I0105597

Next 10 Exits

Reflections on Race and Resilience in Vallejo, California

Elizabeth Ching

Rabbit Roar | San Francisco | 2022

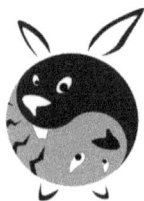

Published by Rabbit Roar
P.O. Box 720177
San Francisco, CA 94172
rabbitroar.com

All text and art copyright © 2022 by Elizabeth Ching
Edited by Valerie Haynes-Perry and Jai Arun Ravine

Book design by Jai Arun Ravine

All rights reserved. No part of this book may be reproduced, scanned, or distrib-
uted in any printed or electronic form without the author's permission. Please
do not participate in or encourage piracy of copyrighted materials in violation
of the author's rights—purchase only authorized editions.

ISBN 978-1-943301-01-0

Advance Praise for *Next 10 Exits*

Dr. Beth Ching sits us upright in the car, rolls down the windows, and urges us to pay attention as she deftly tells us the stories of her hometown, Vallejo. Without her guidance, we would otherwise know nothing about the rich and varied cultural and racial lives that exist beyond the freeway exits demarcating the segregated neighborhoods of this demographically diverse city. The ride through these pages is sprinkled with Dr. Ching's reconstruction of her own family's evolution in the context of Vallejo's ever-changing race and class composition. Dr. Ching shows her brilliance as a scholar with the details of history, her creativity and originality with the insertion of paintings and poetry, and her ability to sit with the loves and sorrows of family life by sharing those intimacies with us throughout. Thank you, Dr. Ching!
Melanie Tervalon, MD, MPH, co-author of *Cultural Humility vs. Cultural Competence*

This short book is a personal journey from the lens of an "Intra-Asian" Native Vallejoan, an occupational therapist, educator, and author who utilized art, writing, and poetry in reflecting and narrating stories of her family and her beloved city of Vallejo. Her stories showcase the importance of diversity, equity, and inclusion and how resiliency, perseverance, and cultural pride can be expressed toward a path of healing from trauma caused by structural racism, prejudice, and injustice. Very authentic, informative, and speaks from the heart!
Luis Arabit, Occupational Therapy Professor, San Jose State University

Through a creative combination of art, poetry, and storytelling, Dr. Ching paints a powerful picture of her youth in a troubled town - a melting pot of races struggling to coexist. The racism of the 60s and 70s that she portrayed was real, and the hatred ran deep. As the town became more diverse, many still clung to their racist views and some still do. At the same time, others let kindness lead the way to a different perspective. For these people, hatred led to tolerance, which led to acceptance, which led to friendships, and, in some cases, led to a celebration of our different cultures. While racism still exists everywhere and has arguably gotten worse, these positive lessons from a downtrodden town can be a catalyst for understanding, healing, hope, and change.
Mike Coffey, Native Vallejoan, retired telecommunications executive

Contents

Art | **Prose** | *Poetry*

*The number in parentheses indicates the page on which a description for the art piece can be found.

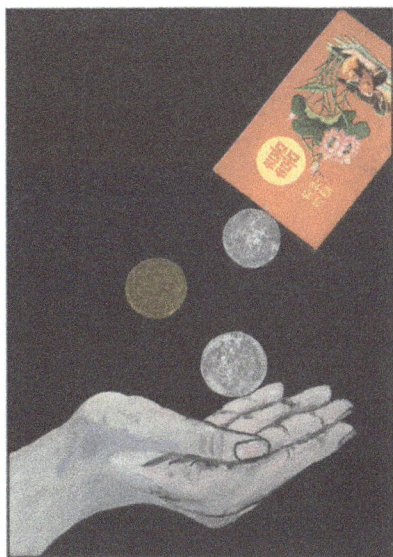

Lucky Money

The red envelope "Licee," given at Lunar New Year and on special occasions like weddings and birthdays, are featured in Chinese culture for luck and prosperity. I painted this piece when I lived in Austin, Texas from 1989 to 1995. Back then, it could be coins and not bills emanating from the red envelope as I remember receiving dollar and fifty-cent pieces back in the day!

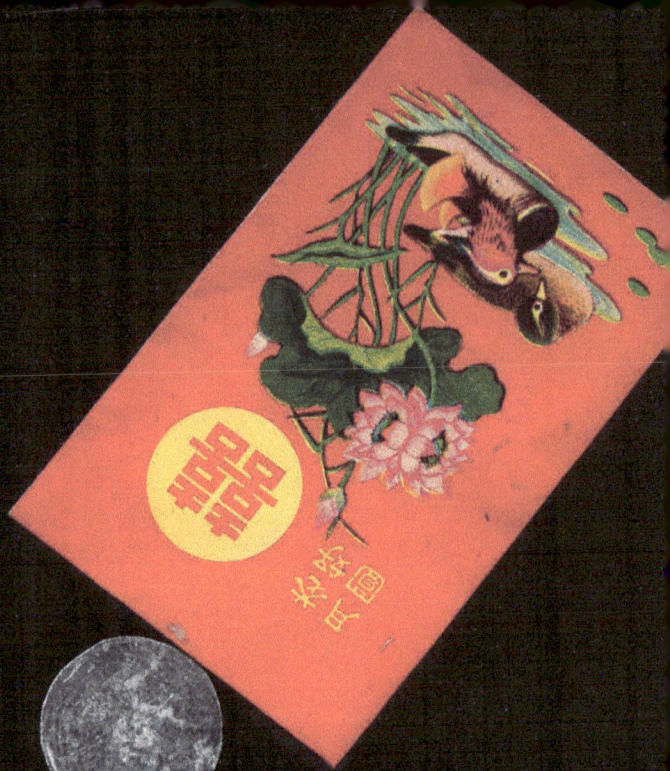

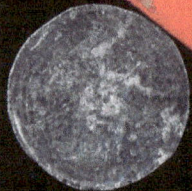

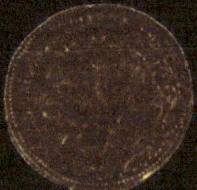

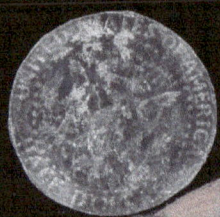

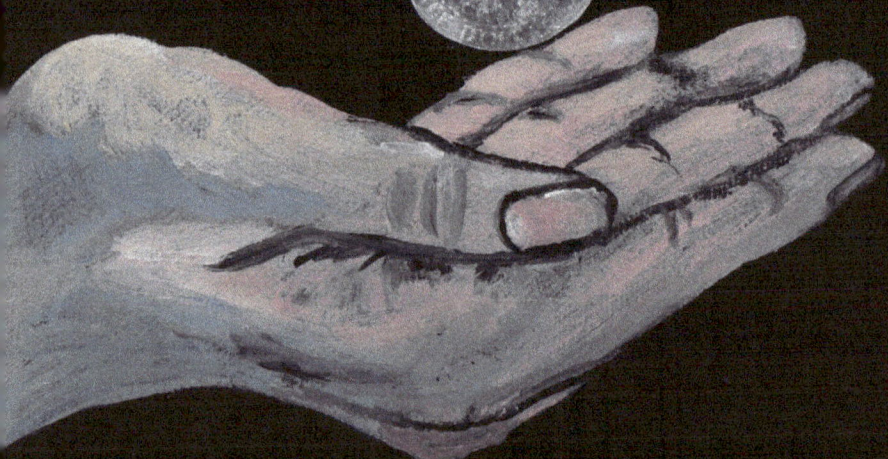

Introduction

According to the 2010 Census, Vallejo, California has the most racially diverse zip codes in the United States. As a Third Generation Korean Chinese American growing up in Vallejo in the 1960s through 1980s and identifying as a Person of Color, my lenses have been shaped by both race and resilience. The now-defunct Mare Island Naval Shipyard brought good-paying work to Vallejo during World War II; this was the reason so many different racial and ethnic groups worked and lived in this small city, current population 122,000.

As a health professional and professor, I have learned about adverse childhood experiences or ACES; that is, early childhood trauma can influence an individual's overall health during that person's lifetime. Vallejo has had three hospitals since the early 20th century. Because of the military presence, physical rehabilitation through Kaiser Hospital has been historic. Since the closing of the Naval Shipyard, hospitals have become the largest employers in Vallejo.

The flipside of trauma can be healing or trauma-informed art. Ernest J. Gaines, the author of *The Autobiography of Miss Jane Pittman*, lived much of his life in Vallejo. Perhaps that is why so many hip-hop artists like E-40, Baby Bash, SOB x RBE, R&B artist H.E.R., plus athletes like C.C. Sabathia, C.J. Anderson, and Natalie Coughlin are Vallejoans.

"Strength through Diversity" is on a plaque at the Vallejo Naval and Historical Museum, yet our current society is much more segregated than during my youth. The ten exits in Vallejo are memory markers of the intersections of race and resilience among the four racial groups, each of which are almost equally divided to comprise approximately 25% of Vallejo: African American, Asian American and Pacific Islander, Latinx, and White populations.

If Vallejo is a microcosm of the U.S. because of its racial diversity, what lessons can we learn about how to affect systemic change to structural racism? How can we reduce health disparities and work toward health equity for all? Through my own personal lenses as a Native Vallejoan, health care practitioner and professor, diversity trainer, and artist, I want to use the mediums of trauma and cultural pride to produce the art of healing. Come with me on my journey through the next 10 exits.

Rust Belt Town

My hometown of Vallejo, California has been in the news lately, but not for pretty reasons. The police murdered another young brother of color this month. This time he was a young Latinx man named Sean Monterrosa, kneeling on the ground to surrender with a hammer in his pocket, and the cop shot him through his windshield.

The byline usually states that the city is located in the San Francisco Bay Area. While technically true, the City of Vallejo is 30 miles northeast of San Francisco and might as well be 3,000 miles away, if you know the history of my hometown. The "Rust Belt" usually refers to Midwestern cities that have lost well-paying manufacturing work, but Vallejo is a Rust Belt city on the West Coast.

I was born in 1962 and grew up in this working-class city. I am a Third Generation Korean and Chinese American and the youngest of five children. Both of my sorely-missed parents are deceased. My father Herbert worked for over 50 years in the one-industry town at Mare Island Naval Shipyard. It employed women and People of Color during its heyday in the 1940s and during World War II.

Before I was born, my family lived in Floyd Terrace, government housing known to many of us from working-class backgrounds as "The Projects." In 1956 when my brother Matthew was born, my family moved to Magazine Street, which you may recognize if you have listened to hip hop in the last couple of decades—it is the same street referred to by E-40.

I am an occupational therapist and a professor. I jokingly tell students that my claim to fame is that I am more of an "O.G." than E-40, except by virtue of the fact that I have never been an "Original Gangster," but am simply older than him. My mother Marguerite, a homemaker, told us that the White residents of the neighborhood we moved to, which ironically happens to be named "Beverly Hills," did not succeed in keeping our family out. We were the first non-White family to move there. White homeowners circulated a petition to prevent us from moving into a prefabricated house, which was $10,000 in 1956 and was what my family could afford. The White residents did not want an Asian family "integrating" the neighborhood.

My father was briefly enlisted in the Army, but he said he was discharged because he had flat feet. He moved from San Francisco's Chinatown to Vallejo, along with my mother, who was born in Reedley, a small farming town in the Central Valley. To support his growing family, my father worked the following three jobs:

1) stocker in a small Chinese grocery store
2) gas station attendant (in the days of full-service)
3) apprentice as a shipbuilding electrical mechanic, which eventually progressed into full-time work

Both of my parents had a high school education, yet Vallejo offered my father gainful employment in well-paying industrial work—just like thousands of African Americans from the South, Filipinos born in the U.S. or in the Philippines, Mexican Americans, and Whites from states like Oklahoma—until Mare Island closed in 1996. The rest is well documented: the city went bankrupt, the school district was taken over by the State, and economic scarcity, unemployment, crime, and violence plagued this suburban North Bay City.

Like many families of color, ours experienced trauma in the form of my eldest brother Kenneth dying at the age of 29 from alcoholism. In retrospect, I had a strong inclination to enter the health professions and benefited by being the youngest where another brother, Ernest, helped me navigate college. Ernest taught U.S. History and Geography among many other courses at Vallejo High School for over 30 years and retired in June 2016. Ernest remarked that "Vallejo was like the 'Rust

Belt'"—people had to work together and occupy the same spaces during the war effort of the 1940s. In his time at Vallejo High, the students were from the lowest socioeconomic groups in the city. Ernest noted that students were more racially segregated than how we both grew up in the 1960s and 1970s, because of private and charter schools siphoning off the more affluent students.

Because Ernest taught several generations of Vallejoans, whenever we go anywhere in Vallejo together, my brother is like a hometown celebrity. "Hi, Mr. Ching!" his former students shout across restaurants, hospitals, or stores. I spoke with him last year about how hopeless I was feeling after reading of the 2019 killing by police of Willie McCoy, who was a 20-year-old African American rapper full of potential and promise. Ernest replied, "I remember him—he was not my student but I saw him on the Vallejo High campus and he was very courteous, respectful, and sharp." We have to "size someone up" quickly. You see, coming from Vallejo from a working-class, person-of-color perspective, as teachers or therapists, we both need to size up a person's character in a short time frame. If students tell me over the phone that they need to be absent from class, I can usually tell just by the timbre of their voices whether the absence is for a legitimate reason—much like as a parent, I know if my son really needs to miss school or not. Ernest bears witness to the waste of this young man's life cut short. Even though we did not know him, we *saw* him.

Now I live with my husband and son Antonio in Oakland, California. (My son is a proud Oaklander.) My husband was born in Laredo, Texas, which was listed in the 2010 census as the least diverse city in the U.S., with the homogeneous population being 98.9% Mexican or Mexican American, given that it is on the southern border with Mexico. My son and I trade good-natured attributes of our respective hometowns. Oakland and Vallejo share similar Great Migration patterns with African Americans; my sister Miriam was the first in my family to move to Oakland in the late 1960s and she commented then that "Oakland is like a Big Vallejo," meaning that the demographics of the two cities were very similar.

Oakland has not been a military or one-industry town like Vallejo. Upon more scrutiny, I have come to realize that it must mean something for Vallejo to have a conservative White analyst like Ed Rollins, as well as the recent Grammy award winner H.E.R., also known as Gabrielle Wilson, who identifies as African American and Filipina and is known for her soulful music. Can you see the spectrum of people from all walks of life that hail from this former Rust Belt of the Bay, the City of Vallejo?

The original people of Vallejo are the Miwok, Suisunes, and Patwin Native Americans. According to the Vallejo Naval and Historical Museum, General Mariano Guadalupe Vallejo was the Mexican military officer for whom the city was named in 1853. The City of Vallejo's website states that their motto is "Vallejo—City of Opportunity." My question is, for whom? As a health professional and educator, I must ask the question: "How can we raise everyone up?" Young people use the medium of hip hop to speak their truths; wasn't Willy McCoy striving to use his life challenges to make art? Isn't this exactly what I say to middle and high school youth of color? I say this to inspire them to think about getting into the health professions. I encourage them to use resiliency and make something positive out of trauma. As the youth say when something is obviously wrong and unjust, "DAMN."

A Note on the Art and Poetry

The art in this book was mainly done either when I was in high school, after starting my first job upon graduating from college, or while I was living in Austin, Texas. I now realize I used the medium of art to deal with challenges or trauma at key junctures of my journey, sprinkled with cultural pride, to begin the process of the lifelong art of healing and growing. The poetry is more recent than the art as I have only included poems that were not previously published in anthologies. Writing has been cathartic for me in these days of the world-wide pandemic, systemic racism, and generalized grief.

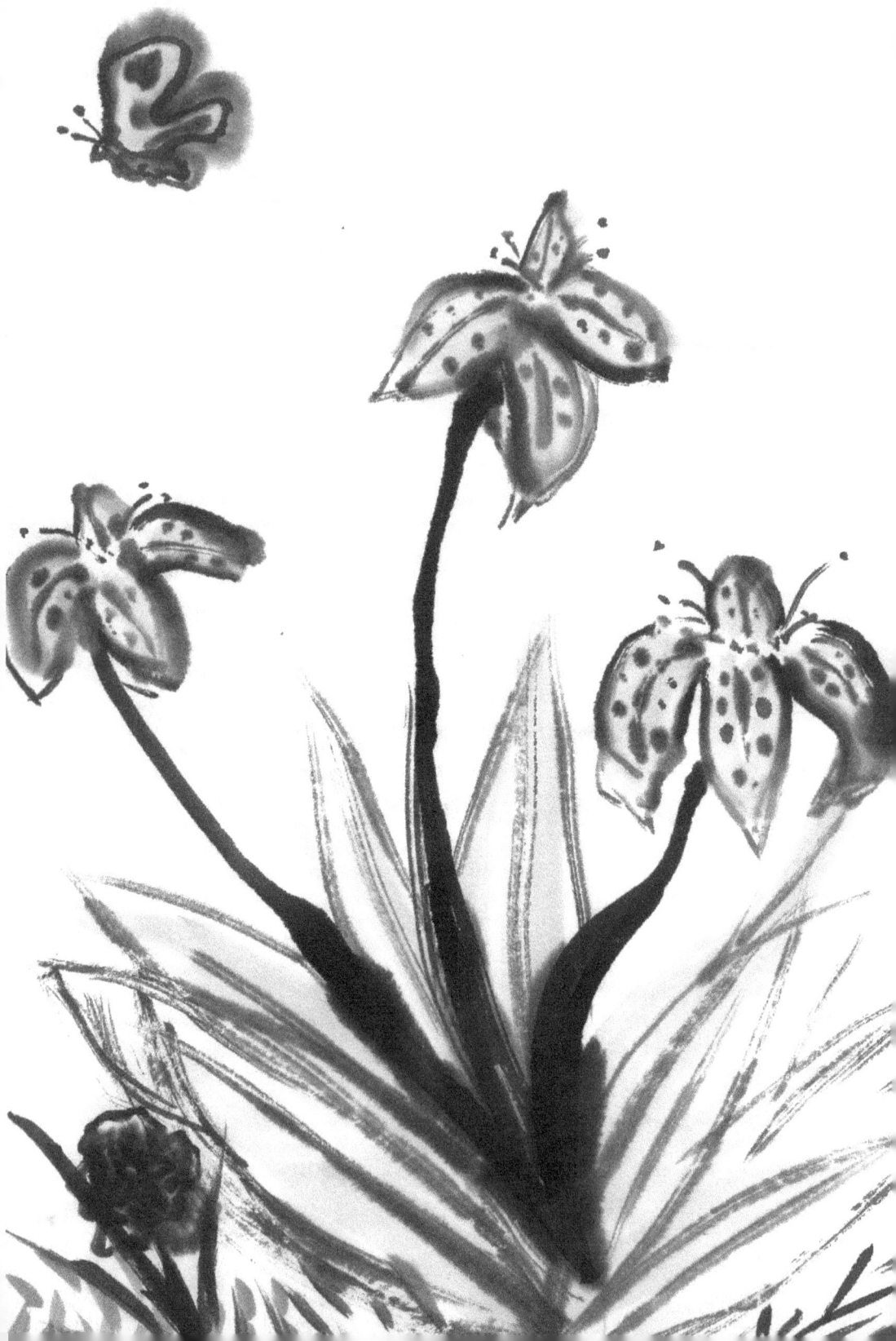

Exit 1 >>> Sonoma Boulevard: South Vallejo

This first exit introduces South Vallejo, which is right after the Carquinez Strait Bridge. South Vallejo was home to one of the early, small mom-and-pop Chinese markets. This exit is devoted to Vallejoans with Chinese heritage.

Gee's Market

We almost lived on Lemon Street in South Vallejo where Filipino and Black families resided in the 1950s, but my parents decided on Magazine Street instead. I remember my father driving us to a tiny Chinese market he called "Gee's" off Sonoma Boulevard. My mother would buy a small rectangle off a gigantic chunk of tofu from a large ice cream freezer-type vat, where tofu swam in its own juices. I detested tofu as a child when my mother cooked it, because it tasted sour and had the odor of old socks. As an adult, I realized that the tofu was not fresh by the time she cooked it; tofu is rather bland and is supposed to take the flavor of the ingredients with which it is cooked. That tofu had to last a long time, given that she would not want to use it all up in one sitting. My mother had a rule—if you did not like her food, you would go to bed hungry. I reserved bitter melon dishes for going to bed with my stomach growling, but tofu was a close second in that contest; I put it in a rolled-up napkin and fed it to our watchdog when no one was looking.

Back then, there were very few places to buy Chinese groceries. There was not an Asian-Latin aisle at the supermarket back in the day. Even getting long-grain white rice was an adventure, as my father would have to make the 40 mile-long trek to San Francisco (S.F.) Chinatown to buy a 50-pound bag of rice. Besides himself and my mother, he had to feed five children. My dad was born in S.F. Chinatown, but he was no longer a "City Slicker," as Vallejo had turned him into a "Country Boy." He was raised by his siblings because he was the youngest and his parents died when he was a child. Herbert Haw Ching, or "Herb" as he was affectionately known by his co-workers, had tuberculosis as a child because of living in crowded conditions in Chinatown. My father recounted fondly his common childhood science experiment of poking toothpicks into a potato, suspending it halfway in a cup of water, and placing it on the windowsill of his family's small apartment. I can still picture my father's wide smile when he noted his pleasant surprise of seeing roots grow in the cup's murky water. This act was the beginning of my father's green thumb. Later, his summer garden on Magazine Street was well known in the neighborhood for its tomatoes and zucchini on one side of the house; loquats, nectarines, peaches, apricot, and plum trees grew on the other side. This former Chinatown kid was living his best life with the luxury of a half-acre of land in Vallejo.

Because we were a working-class family and my father was a "home-body," as my mother called him, we never had a brand new car. We had a lot of "jalopies" though, which were standard drives, not automatics. At the time, I am sure my parents were so stressed, but I have fond childhood memories of getting out of the car to "Push!" That is, we had car problems and our worst fears were being stuck on the Bay Bridge on our way to see family, or going shopping for a large rice sack in S.F. Chinatown. "Gun it!" my father would shout to my brother, to try and start the ignition while not "flooding" the engine. We would park facing down on steep city hills and have bricks in front of both the driver and passenger tires as added security to the emergency brake. One family member would carefully remove the bricks and get in the car while another would drive, take off the emergency brakes, and coast until the ignition turned over. Nothing in these cars was automatic; that is, if you wanted the windows open, you had to roll them down with a crank. Those were the days of bucket seats, no seat belts, and definitely no child car seats. It is a wonder that I am still alive to tell the tale. To this day, I have never owned a new car; I have owned next-to-new cars. My take-away from my father was to avoid debt and pay cash whenever possible.

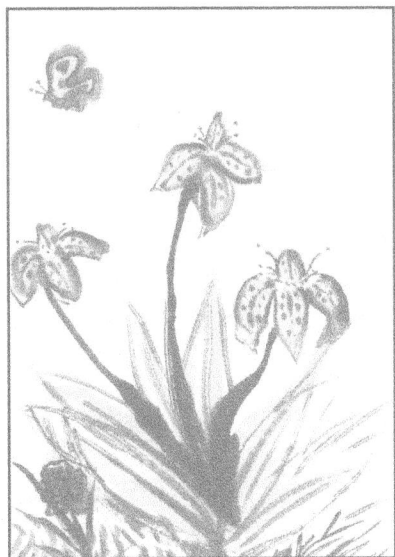

Butterfly and Lilies

"Chinese Brush Painting" was the name of the El Cerrito Adult Education art class when I painted this piece in the mid-1980s. I wanted to explore a new medium with the black ink and traditional Chinese painting. At the time, I was renting a room and living by myself after college. I also had my first job as an occupational therapist in an acute psychiatric setting. I had three positions within a span of five years, and felt as free as a butterfly to go from flower to flower, or from job to job.

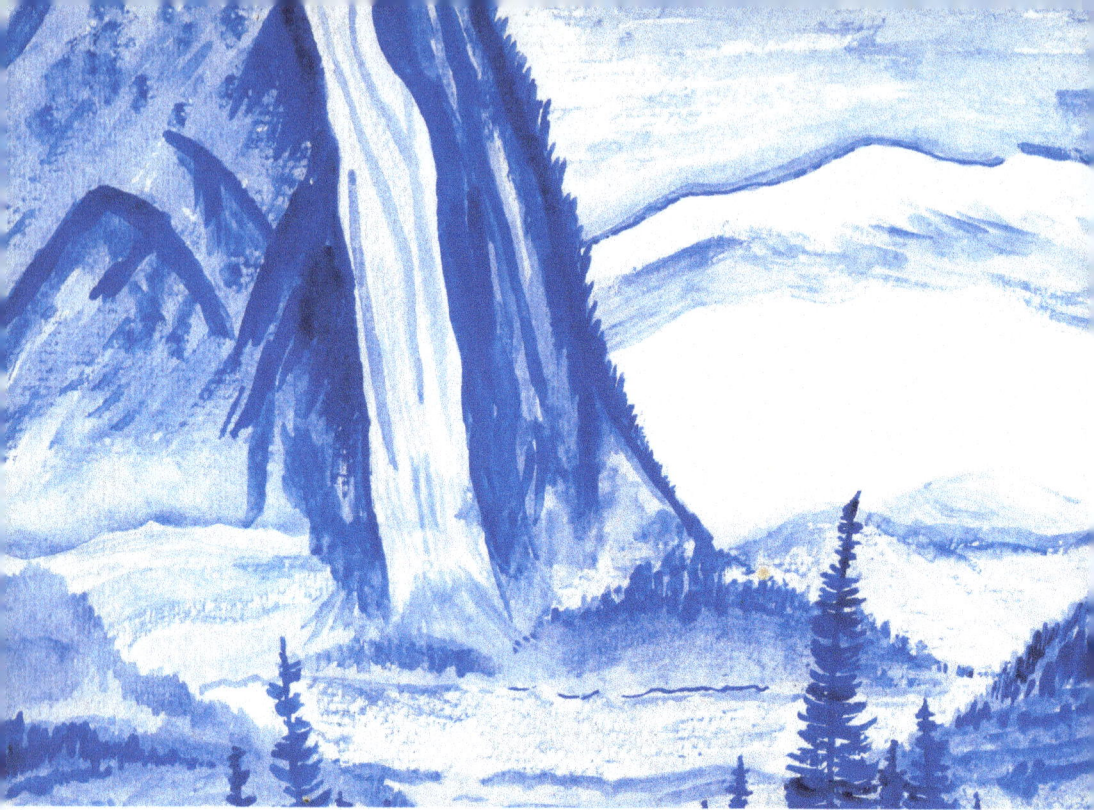

Watercolor Waterfall

This watercolor painting was in my mind's eye of a Yosemite waterfall. Being Asian American and growing up near the Pacific Ocean, I realized that water is always calming to me and I like to live near it even if I rarely visit the beach—it is comforting to know a body of water is close by. I lived in El Cerrito, California when I painted this landscape. "El Cerrito" is Spanish for "the little hill," so my little hill of a waterfall is calming, which is probably the same reason workers buy little fountains for their office spaces.

Exit 2 >>> Sequoia Street

This second exit is home to the California State Maritime Academy. It is devoted to Vallejoans with Pacific Islander heritage.

Maritime Academy

The California State University (CSU) Maritime Academy is off this exit. In addition to being a "Rust Belt Town," Vallejo is also a "Port of Entry"; it is home to the Carquinez Straits where waterways, as well as freeways and intersections, meet. This CSU campus has the largest number of Pacific Islander students in the entire CSU system. Tongans, Samoans, Hawaiians, and Pacific Islanders were part of the Vallejoan Family of Nations, given the racial diversity of Vallejo. Growing up, there was a Guamanian family on the same block as mine; some Guamanians refer to themselves as Chamorros, the indigenous people of Guam. There is no denying the connection of Pacific Islanders to the ocean.

The CSU Maritime Academy's motto is "Ready to Work or Fight," which is fitting. California State Governor Gavin Newsom declared that the CSU Maritime Academy would be the first CSU to open up after the COVID-19 "Shelter-in-Place" orders were relaxed. So much depends on graduates entering the shipping industry, and the maritime impact on the overall health of the economy.

Port of Entry and Historical Trauma

Vallejo is a crossing of land, waterways, freeways, and places to gather, but also places to make a quick escape. This history has made Vallejo home to historical trauma related to violence. In the 1960s, Lake Herman and Blue Rock Springs were waterways not far from the Sequoia exit; they were part of or within the city limits of Vallejo, but also the settings of the Zodiac Killer murders. Vallejo, as a port of call, has seen its share of drugs and other substances of choice, such as alcohol in the early 1900s, or cocaine in the 1970s and 1980s. Alcohol, drugs, prostitution, violence, and other harms have often gone unaddressed in Vallejo, because it is seen as a suburb of San Francisco. Yet, Vallejo suffers from "urban issues" associated with drugs, gangs, and violence related to these underground activities. Robberies have occurred with more frequency since Mare Island closed, as there is no major source of industry left in the city. When there are problems with the Bay Area Rapid Transit (BART) or the subway train, commuters return to taking the ferry from Vallejo to the Embarcadero in San Francisco.

My brother Kenneth succumbed physically to acute liver failure and jaundice as a result of alcoholism. In my view, emotionally, he died of internalized oppression and a form of self-hatred. These resulted from existing in a society where he was not seen as a handsome, strong Asian man with inherent worth and dignity. People said Kenny looked like Bruce Lee (if Bruce were also part Korean) with thick black hair, a wide chest and a small waist. By all accounts, he was a child with an abundance of energy and spirit that caused him to "get a whipping" several times a day. As the eldest son of an Asian family, I believe he was always striving to do well in the dominant society that never accepted him. I was ten years younger than him and the "baby" of the family, so he doted on me, which meant I escaped having a difficult and complicated relationship with him, as he could be a con artist. For many People of Color, substance use and abuse are a form of self-medication, which can lead to self-euthanization.

My Auntie and Native Hawaiians

California is the closest "mainland" state to Hawaii. Thus, it is easy to see why many Native Hawaiians would rather live near the Pacific Ocean in a climate and culture more similar to the islands, instead of other states where this is not the case. Before the Oakland Raiders moved to Las Vegas, many Hawaiians chose the Raiders as their NFL team because the State of Hawaii does not have its own.

One side of my family has some members who settled in Hawaii. My "Auntie" is a Native Hawaiian; she is not technically my aunt but is married to my cousin. In fact, she met my cousin through a 12-Step program. When we went to visit her and my cousin, she said that she wanted to take my family to the Bishop Museum, which showcases Native Hawaiian history and culture in Honolulu. While I was pulling out my wallet, she told the cashier that because she was a Native Hawaiian who did not pay an entrance fee, as her family we should be admitted for free, too. Lo and behold, we all entered the Bishop Museum free of charge! The Aloha Spirit is definitely a reality.

There is family through blood lines and there is definitely family through choice. When my son was nine years old, my Auntie taught him about making music with the "hands-on" drum exhibit. She encouraged him through example and by telling him that he had a "gift" with the beat. She is a survivor and someone who reminds me of the power of kinship, kindness, and loyalty. In many ways, I think people who make it through hard times in Vallejo carry that Aloha Spirit, even though they are not from Hawaii, because of the influence of Pacific currents gathering there.

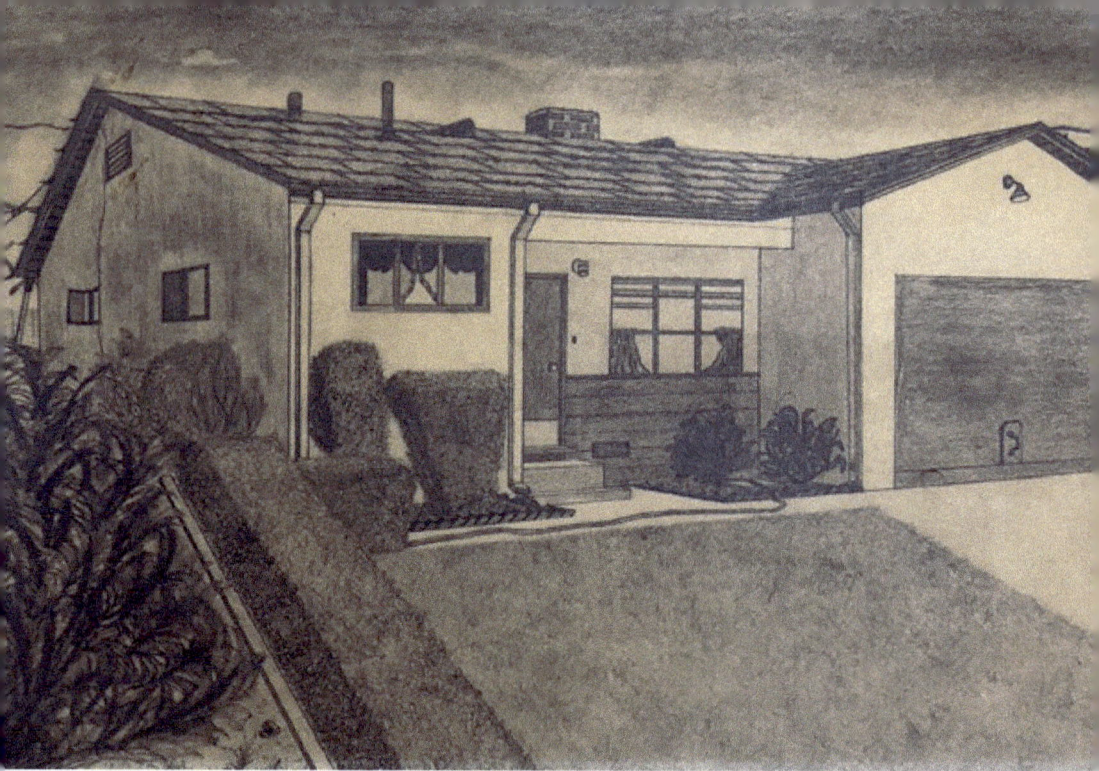

Magazine Street

I drew this pencil sketch of my former home in high school to illustrate perspective. My mother was an amazing person struggling with an untreated psychiatric diagnosis, yet she raised five children mainly by herself, as my father did not take on many of the childrearing duties. My father had an undiagnosed learning disorder. In retrospect, I had a strong inclination to enter the health professions, and my practice setting is mental health and brain injury. In my first position in Occupational Therapy (OT) at an acute psychiatric hospital, a social worker said, "Beth, most people that work in psychiatric hospitals have been doing this type of work all their lives, but now they are getting paid for it."

Exit 3 >>> Magazine Street

This third exit speaks to my childhood home on Magazine Street. It is devoted to Vallejoans with Korean heritage.

Outside City Limits

The sidewalk stopped right before our house on Magazine Street. Our home was the first house outside the city limit. Being in the city and outside the city is a metaphor for being both Chinese and Korean. My father's motto was "Don't make waves," which symbolizes the Chinese harmony virtue. My mother's signature description of a Korean trait was that there were some people who had a "Kimchee Temper," or were quick to anger. Because we lived in Northern California, we were closest to my father's Ching side of the family. If we had grown up in Southern California like my cousins in Pico Rivera, we would have been closest to my mother's Yoon side. "IntraAsian" is how I describe the kind of Asian I am. I am not mixed heritage per se, as Korean and Chinese are both Asian nationalities. However, they both have very distinct languages, expressions, and cultures.

Take how spirituality is expressed. During the spring, my father would observe what he called "Hong Ching," to honor ancestors by going to the Chinese Cemetery in Colma to bow three times, light incense, and offer the deceased their favorite foods. There were endless arguments by my parents because my father would bring back the delicious food for the family, and my mother would say we could not eat it because it was offered to "false gods and idolatry." You see, she was the youngest daughter and "a pastor's kid" who gave up religion but then came back to it so she could bring up her five children religiously. When she was a rebellious teen, she confessed that she "played hooky from school and smoked cigarettes," because it was too much pressure to be good as the child of a Presbyterian theologian and diplomat.

My mother was born in the Central Valley in Reedley, California. My grandfather came to the U.S. in the early 1900s and would go back and forth to Korea to organize and fight for independence from Japan.

Meanwhile, my grandmother mainly raised 11 children on her own, losing two to malnutrition, another to suicide, and another to a farming vehicle accident. My understanding is that "Han" speaks to Korea's collective grief after being colonized and then split into two.

For many years, only my father was allowed to eat the "cha-sui bau" (barbeque pork buns) and little custards because he was "a heathen" according to my mother! Finally, after much turmoil, my mother met with her Nazarene pastor who told her that God would be accepting of peace between a husband and wife. After the pastor's blessing, my mother prayed or "said grace" before allowing us to scarf down the food that came from S.F. Chinatown once a year.

Someone once asked me what the "Nazarene" faith was. I said it was like being a Baptist but even less fun, as we were not allowed to dance because it was "too sexual." You can tell that the Nazarene church where we were members had mainly White congregants. Contrary to leading *to* sex, going to high school dances was a way of postponing sex as far as I could tell. My mother sent me to a Nazarene summer camp in the Santa Cruz mountains. I was the only Person of Color, and church kids could be so mean and cliquey. At the campfire, I learned a few more songs, like "If You're Happy and You Know It" and "Bringing in the Sheaves," besides "This Little Light of Mine," and I ate s'mores for the first time.

When my parents were alive, they both contributed to the war effort as my father was an electrical mechanic building ships and my mother was a homemaker. I remember her recounting how she would draw lines with a pen onto the back of her bare legs "so it would look like I was wearing stockings." In truth, she was not wearing stockings because nylon was used only for the war effort, rather than nonessentials like pantyhose. They also lived through the Great Depression, so I learned to cook, knit, and sew. My father's garden was well-known in my working-class neighborhood. In hindsight, my siblings and I learned skills which many People of Color hone—how to become more self-sufficient for surviving hard times.

Being part of at least two cultures allows one to see different sides. You can be at peace with what might seem like contradictions, such as being in the country part of the City of Vallejo.

Our family home was sold some years ago. When I passed by the house, I did not see it as fully as before, because the owners had built a lovely fence. My father had built a fence several times, but we would wake up in the night hearing crashes from the bottom of two hills, coming either from Gilcrest Street or cars barreling down Magazine Street. My dad gave up and just left the fence posts.

Chinese Korean American

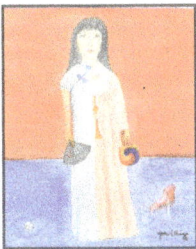

I did this watercolor painting when I lived in Austin, Texas in the early 1990s to try getting out of my comfort zone of sketching and acrylic painting. The left side is a Chinese cheung-sam dress and the right side is a Korean han-bok dress, depicting being IntraAsian or having two distinct Asian identities. The high-top basketball shoes are what I used when I was on my high school badminton team, and the baseball represents "America's Sport." I love watercolor paintings at museums; however, I realized I like to be in control of the medium and it was challenging to "let it go" as watercolor flows where it wants to. When I used watercolor in high school art class, I only used it for a background, not the main imagery. As a teacher, I like to have control in the classroom.

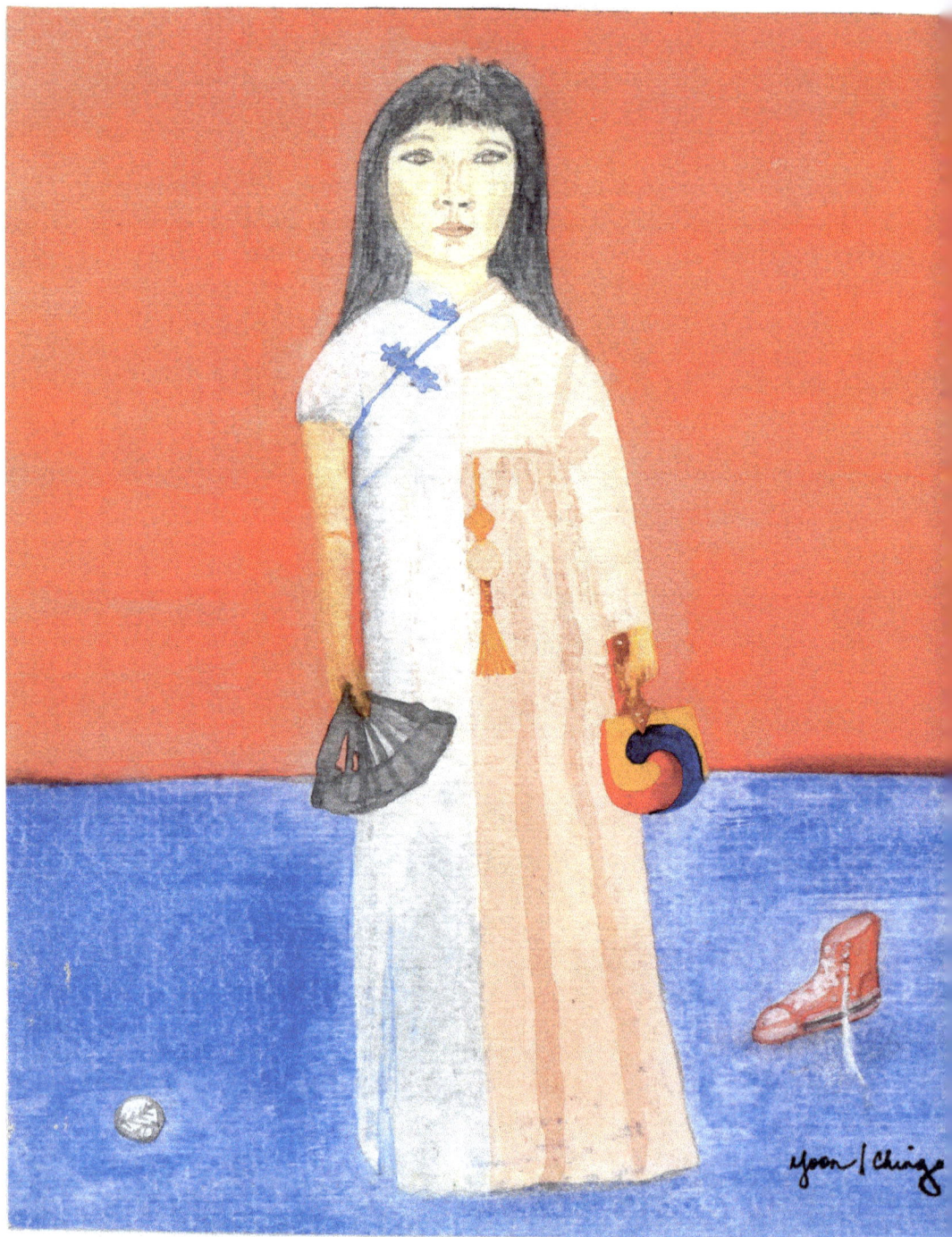

Magnolias and Persimmons

Magnolias were one of my mother's favorite flowers, and like many other Koreans, she enjoyed persimmons with the tart but sweet taste that also perfectly describes my mother's temperament. In the following poem, I was getting perspective on her birthplace of Reedley, California, which is a very agricultural Central-California town where my grandfather settled. It was highly unusual to be a Korean living in the U.S. at the start of the 1900s; my grandfather was among those early Korean settlers and patriots honored for their sacrifices for the U.S. and for Korea.

I did not want to say that I was really there for you, Ma.
Honoring ten Korean patriots was the occasion.
Grandpa Pyong Koo Yoon
Figured prominently—
You would be so proud.
Truth be told, it was all about
Seeing where you were born—
Central California, Reedley, Fruit Bowl
November 13, 2010
So close to your birthday
November 16, 1925
It all made sense—how you were a
Farm girl who loved buttermilk,
Rhubarb, bacon, lemon meringue
That is what finally got you in the end,
Arteriosclerosis
When I looked across the street
From the Memorial Monuments,
From the Independence Gate,
From the American and Korean Flags,
I saw you—a rose of a different color
bordering the house with the persimmons
and the neighboring house with the magnolias
Rest in Peace, Minnie Marguerite.

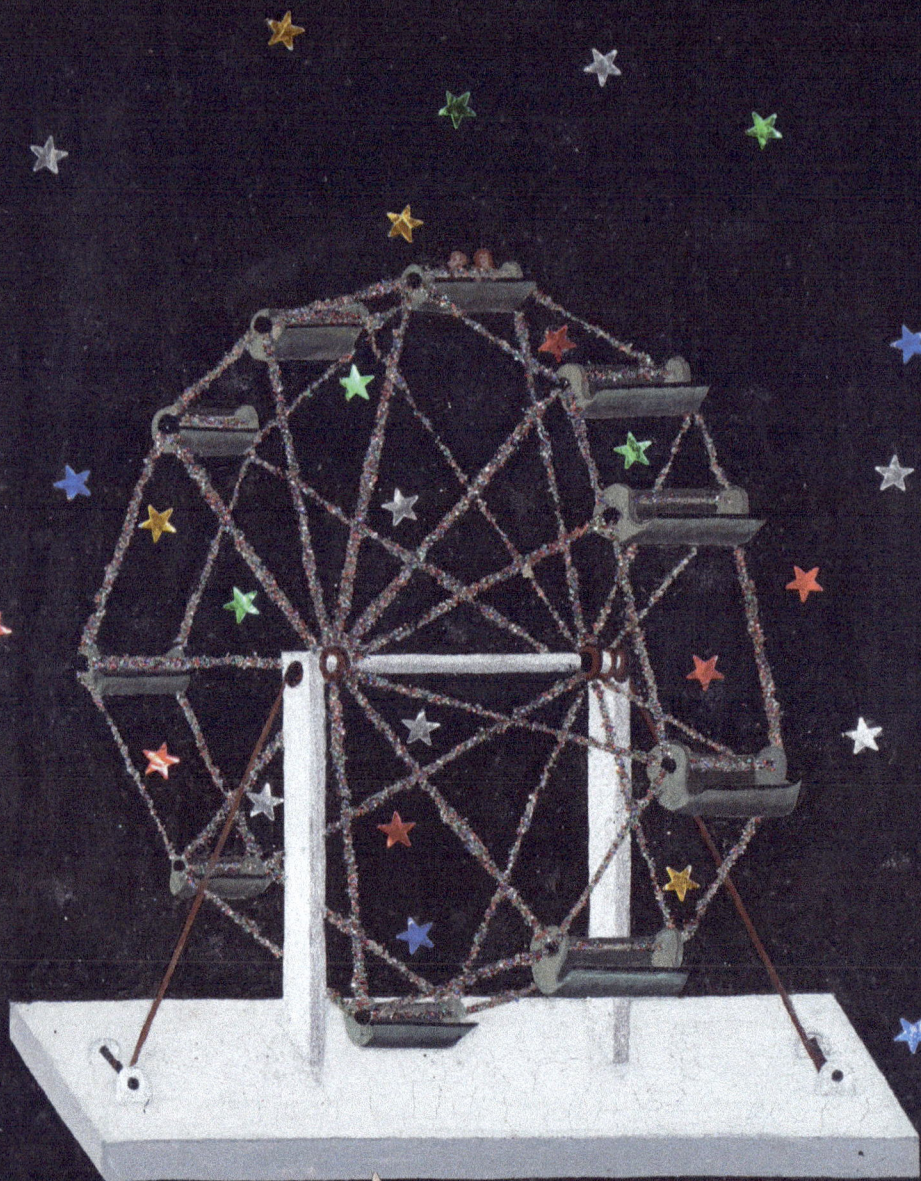

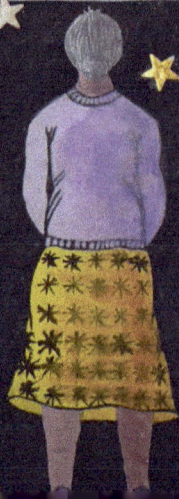

Exit 4 >>> Benicia / Curtola Parkway

This fourth exit is in Vallejo but leads to the City of Benicia. It is devoted to Vallejoans with Native American or Indigenous heritage.

Benicia State Park

I can smell the ocean and hear the lap of waves as I look for pretty pebbles in my mind's eye at Benicia State Park. The City of Benicia was the state capital only once, but Vallejo was the state capital twice before eventually losing to Sacramento in the 1800s. The City of Benicia was named after the wife of General Mariano Vallejo. The leader of the Suisunes, a Patwin People, was Sem-Yeto, who was renamed Chief "Solano" and befriended General Vallejo.

Glen Cove is an area in Vallejo that is right before Benicia. The Shell Mounds in Glen Cove are sacred to Native people. They had to fight to retain the Shell Mounds as the Greater Vallejo Recreation District (GVRD) had planned to expand portions of the park to build restrooms on the sacred site. In reality, this is where the origin story of the City of Vallejo began, which is also based on historical trauma to Native Americans. The school mascot for Vallejo High had been "The Apaches," but was finally changed to "Red Hawks" in 2014. If there were no Native Americans in Vallejo asking for a change, the offensive name would still be used to this day. Indigenous people are staying strong in response to generations of injustice.

The Longest Walk and Recycling

"Do we have any wool blankets we can donate to 'The Longest Walk'?" my brother Ernest asked my parents in 1978. The five-month walk from San Francisco to Washington, D.C. brought attention to Native American issues, and I suspect the march made a stop in Vallejo because of some prominent Native American organizers from Vallejo. I remember thinking that I hoped the blankets we donated did not have any moth-eaten holes or were too raggedy in general. We always had old wool blankets that would still retain warmth when wet but were so heavy, I struggled as a child to even toss and turn at night. Donations from my household were well-intentioned but had seen better days, as they had been exchanged at least five times before I received the "hand-me-downs."

In my family, we recycled for as long as I can remember. We would use the same bathtub full of water from person to person so much, I often said I did not know if I was cleaner when I got in the tub or when I got out. To this day, I cannot shake the habit of melding the tiniest bit of bath bar soap to the new bath bar soap, or adding the smallest amount of water to the ketchup bottle to get the last plop of sauce to slide out onto my fries. We knew others had it harder than we did, and we always identified with marginalized groups.

Confrontation Strategy

Growing up in Vallejo, I learned not to "start something." My mother taught us to "turn the other cheek," which was her biblical way of telling us not to fight. However, she did tell us that we were allowed to "hit back" if someone else started hitting us first. I always tried to avoid the call of "there's going to be a fight after school" by taking the opposite route from the fight home.

This confrontation strategy has served me well as a relative newcomer to academia. A few years into my current position at a health science university, a colleague disagreed with me on a subject by e-mailing me two journal articles that backed up her opinion, which she told me I "should read." I thanked her for the resources and sent her two journal articles that backed up my opinion and told her to read them also. This was the academic equivalent of a street fight where she gave me the finger, and I returned the favor by giving her two fingers in the guise of two peer-reviewed journals. I avoid confrontation as much as possible, but sometimes you "have to throw down," otherwise there are those who will take away your power.

I can still smell summer in the reeds and cattails along the trail in Benicia State Park. That gentle fragrance helps me center myself in the midst of those busy intellectualizing their privilege and greed.

Dreams of the Fair

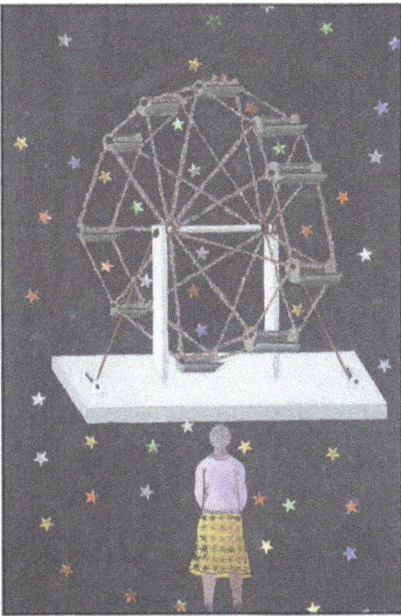

This sparkly acrylic painting with glitter and colored stars was completed in high school. The figure is wistfully looking at the Ferris wheel to convey my desire to go to the fair, which was not guaranteed. Each year in June, the Solano County Fair went on complete with carnival rides, a gem show, a livestock exhibit, corn dogs, and so on. Because of the entrance fee and spending money needed, I was not allowed to go some years, being from a working-class family. One year, my brother Kenneth said, "Here Bethie. Take this money and go to the fair!" I was not expecting to be able to go, so I went with my across-the-street neighbor and had a grand time. When Ken died, that was one of my fondest memories of his generosity and brotherly love.

Elizabeth Ching

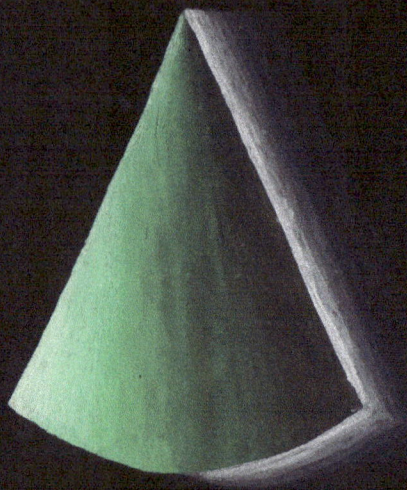

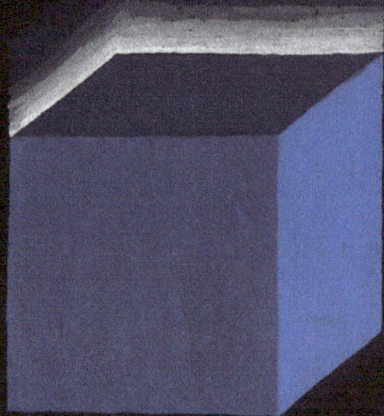

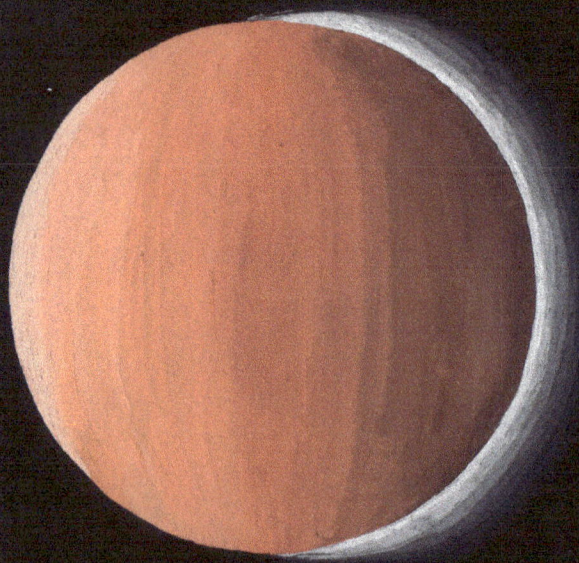

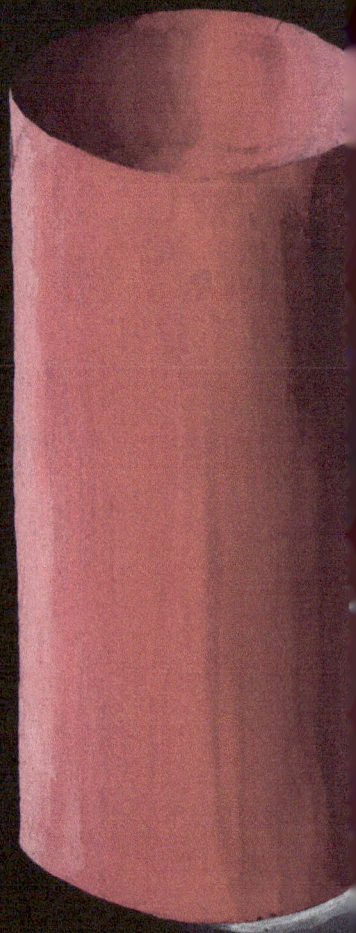

Exit 5 >>> Georgia Street / Central Vallejo

This fifth exit introduces Central Vallejo, which is the home to downtown or "Old Vallejo." The Waterfront is here and so is the Farmer's Market, which is still held on Georgia Street. Vallejoans have been gathering downtown ever since Vallejo became a city.

Gathering Places

The Waterfront is a concrete walkway that runs parallel to the Carquinez Strait and faces Mare Island, which was where the buildings that serviced the naval ships were housed. A cherry bomb almost kissed my achilles heel when we went to the Waterfront to be closer to the fireworks on the Fourth of July in 1971. Mini-explosions were going on all around my nine-year-old self. People from all walks of life gathered downtown for the Fourth of July Fireworks, Farmer's Market, Empress Theatre, and the Army Surplus Store.

I went back recently and was reminded how much of a military presence Vallejo retains, even though Mare Island has been shuttered for decades now. There was a family festival outdoors at the Waterfront with assorted booths of shaved ice, tacos, corn-on-the-cob, lumpia, and hot links. Walking into the children's area, I did a double-take as the fence that blocked off the children's section was spray-painted in a camouflage pattern and bales of hay were stacked so children could turn the corner and shoot each other with lasers. Remember now, I currently live in Oakland, close to people who are attracted to the Bay Area for its progressive political leanings. Nearby Berkeley has face painting and unicorns in the children's area of their street fairs. What a difference 30 miles makes!

In 1970, the John F. Kennedy library opened right across from the Waterfront. I am from one of the Dewey Decimal System generations. The turnstiles at the front entrance of the library would give me a soft thud on my chest, and I would see the newspaper stacks on the right and the reference table directly ahead. The style was modern at the time with high ceilings and abstract art. That building gave my brother Ernest a job and my brother Matthew check-outs of DVDs, and I took naps in the crooks of my elbows there when I was a student at Solano Community College. That place was a sanctuary for folks of all ages, especially the section for children's books on the second floor.

Merrill's Drug Store used to be a favorite destination after church when my father picked us up; he would get cigarettes and allow us kids to get some candy, occasionally. Most of the time we walked home from church, even though our home was miles away. We got away with going only to an hour of Sunday school and could avoid the one-and-a-half-hour Sunday service for adults.

"The Sabbath" was my only half-day off. I had to attend Chinese school on Saturday with my mother at Lincoln Elementary School on Sonoma Boulevard downtown, where parts of Cartoon Network's "Amazing World of Gumball" provide the setting. My poor mother... We both felt like we were dumb because our classmates were children like me, but they already spoke Cantonese and merely came to learn the written Chinese characters or calligraphy. My Mom was "ABK" or an American-Born Korean; her generation was told to assimilate so she only knew a few words of Korean. My father wanted me to learn Chinese even though I could never get the tone right. Go figure—I ended up getting a minor in Spanish and using it to speak with my monolingual Spanish-speaking mother-in-law. I attempted to learn Cantonese again in my twenties; however, shade was cast at me as my Chinese American college room-mate said I sounded like a "faun-yin," also known as a White person, when I tried to speak Chinese.

My mother persuaded us to host our Fourth of July family gatherings. Because my husband is a Tejano, we skip the burgers and hot dogs and have carne asada or fajita, sausage, chicken, grilled vegetables, and beans and rice instead. Oakland used to launch fireworks at the Embarcadero, but this year will be the first Fourth we will not be hosting since 1995.

Basic Shapes

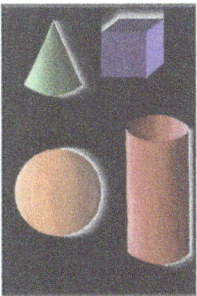

My high school art teacher told us that we could paint almost anything if we mastered painting the four basic (3D) shapes of the sphere, cylinder, cone, and cube. It took quite some time, but I managed to paint the basic shapes. This acrylic painting symbolizes downtown Vallejo as people from all walks of life—all different shapes and sizes—make up the beautiful diversity that is the City of Vallejo.

Elizabeth Ching

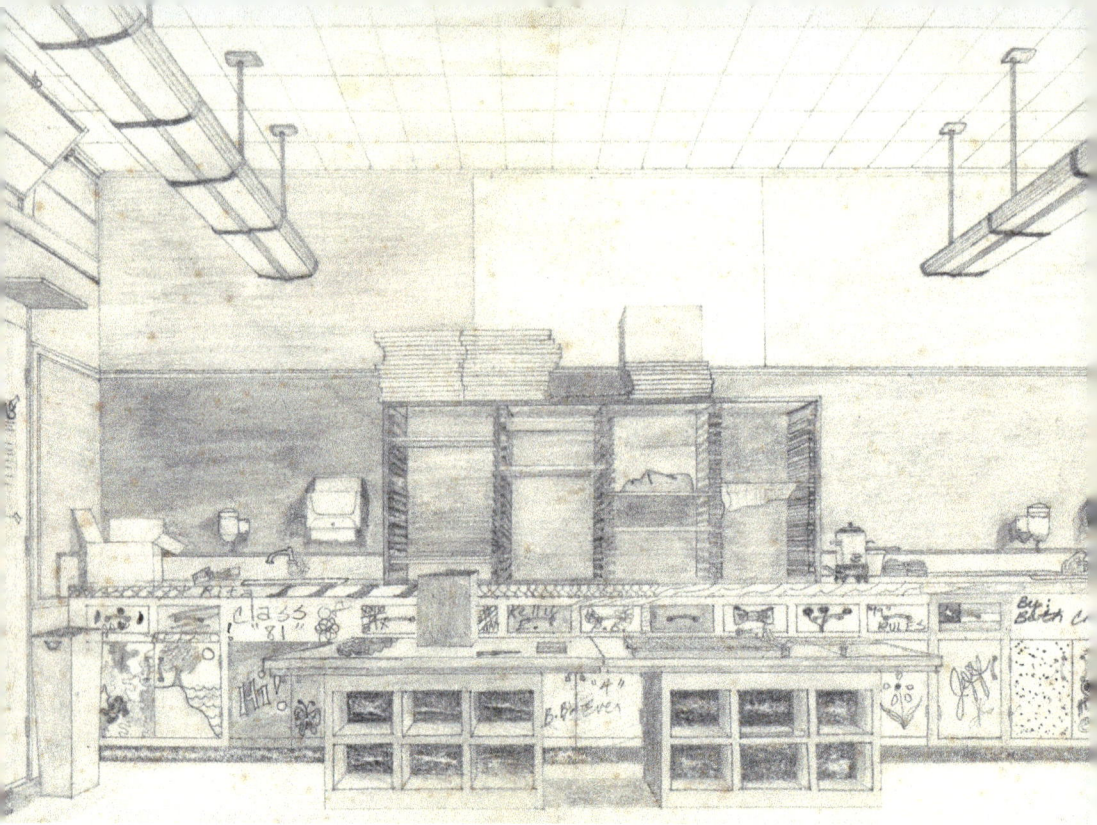

Hogan High Art Room

I graduated Class of 1980 from Hogan High School. This pencil drawing resulted from a senior assignment. We had to draw something with perspective and shading to reflect three-dimensional aspects of the environment to give it depth. Notice the cubby holes where our pieces were placed to dry, and the graffiti on the cupboards being an occupational hazard of the art space with budding artists. This was before liquid soap, so the soap dispenser held white powder that you mixed with water to provide a gravelly hand cleaning experience.

When I was in art class, there would be fights about what music we would listen to, because some White students might want to hear Leonard Skynard and some Black students might want to hear Funkadelic. Somehow, "One Nation Under A Groove" is embedded in my mind as an anthem of the victors of the record player, at least in Art period. Classmates used to smoke weed in the back of the room, but they were very respectful of our wonderful art teacher who was reserved yet totally supportive of us. He himself was a work of art!

Exit 6 >>> Solano Avenue / Springs Road

This sixth exit introduces Springs Road and Solano Avenue, two areas that fed into Hogan High School. It focuses on Vallejoans who identify as White.

Hogan High

This part of town was mainly White in the 1970s, and the "new money" or affluent families lived here. If their high-schoolers were not at a private school like Saint Patrick's (males) or Saint Vincent's (females), they went to the public high school, Hogan Senior High. It was on Rosewood, a street parallel to Springs Road. Hogan High had some racial diversity but was not nearly as diverse as Vallejo High, which had the "old money" at the time. Vallejo High is still the oldest public high school, with a giant century-old-plus redwood tree in the front.

African Americans were bussed into the school from Country Club Crest or North Vallejo to "integrate" Hogan High. If you were not part of the Black-White dichotomy of the U.S. racial spectrum, you faced much bullying. My brother Ernest told us there were "race wars" when he was in junior high in the 1970s. Not long after the Civil Rights Movement, as an Asian American, he had to choose if he was going to be on the "White" side or the "Black" side. He chose Black and never looked back! This is why I bristle when Asians are not included when the term "People of Color" is used.

A lesson learned in high school was that teenagers respected you as a teacher if you were passionate about the subject you taught. Mr. "Biology" taught at Hogan. He was White, wore large horn-rimmed glasses, and ate Chinese food warmed up in Pyrex dishes on Bunsen burners at lunch. He was what my peers called "goofy." Yet he was still a favorite teacher of many students of all ethnicities, because he made biology so fascinating.

After High School

My eldest brother Kenneth died of substance abuse. My middle brother Matthew went into the Army soon after high school as the result of being recruited relentlessly. To this day he smokes menthol cigarettes, which have been highly marketed to African Americans. I believe both of my brothers experienced psychological trauma, which grossly affects communities of color. Wikipedia defines this term as "damage to the mind that occurs as a result of a distressing event."

It seemed off to me that I went to my high school reunion in 2018, which was 38 years since I graduated in 1980; I thought it would be in 2020 for the 40th year. As I write this during the COVID-19 period in 2020, I am glad my classmates decided to do it sooner than later; they said that they wanted to host it because so many of our classmates had already died. I was not shocked, but I was saddened with the realization that Hogan was the more affluent of the two public high schools of the time. Yet and still, I suspect many passed away because of structural racism/social determinants of health/co-morbidities because the hosts of the reunion read off an "In Memoriam" list that was so lengthy, it took my breath away. Most of the classmates' names off the list were African American, and diabetes, high blood pressure, and the life stressors of systemic racism shortens lifespans by decades in worse case scenarios.

Currently, Hogan is no longer a high school, but rather a middle school. One of the few friends from high school with whom I still keep in touch is White. He and I have different political views, but he told me he has always valued "diversity" because he knew what it was like to be the only White person in a group; coming from Vallejo, he felt what it was to be an "outsider." He was the friend who taught me the meaning of the term "Wannabe." That is, he knew he was White and did not try to act like he was not. Coming from our multicultural city, being "fake" or inauthentic was a trait we learned to avoid at an early age.

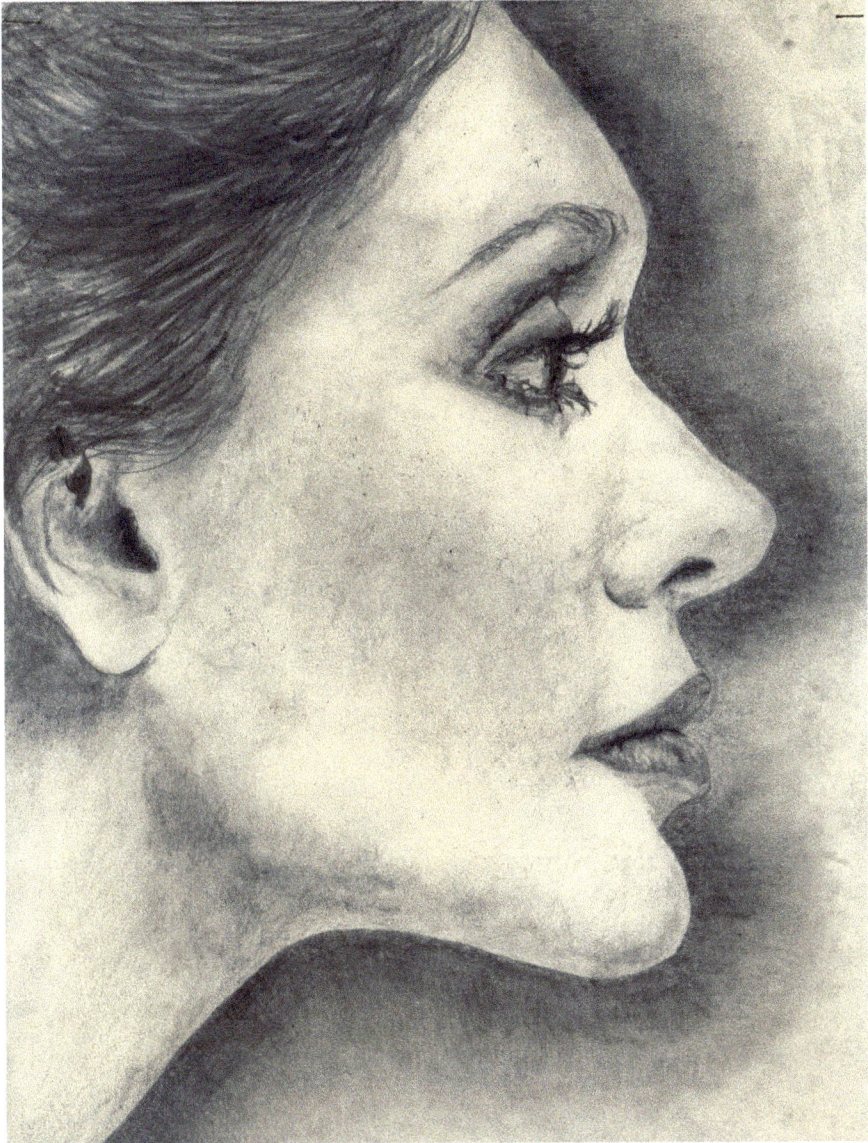

Profile

As a high school art assignment, I had to pick a photo from a magazine to draw a profile. In 1979, many of the magazine ads did not feature People of Color, so I picked this profile of a White woman. The modern-day usage of the word "profile" or "profiling" often does not refer to the dominant culture in the U.S., but rather People of Color, so there is some irony in this pencil drawing.

No Need to Manufacture Soul

This poem was the impetus to write this book. Some things cannot be taught and having "soul" is one of them.

Got triggered again in dance class
You see, been taking what started as a Zumba class has morphed
Into a hip-hop-esque, Afro-Latin dance class
Dance instructor of color mad talented and half my age
But she got to manufacture soul to the mainly White
With a sprinkling of Asian and Latinx sisters
In the rapidly gentrifying
City of Oakland where my son was born 15 years ago.
Me—I'm from Vallejo, California
One-industry, manufacturing, working-class town, Naval Shipyard closed in 1996 then
City went bankrupt, school district taken over by State,
25 miles north of Oakland
But might as well be 2500
Born in 1962 but no need for the instructor to tell me how to say,
"Heeeyyy" when I'm feelin' it.
Only one in class wearing high top basketball shoes
'Cause dancing on hardwood floors just like the Hogan High gym I played
Basketball, badminton, and went to dances
Start moving once the music comes on, no need to wait for directions.
Don't complain when air-conditioning not working 'cause
It's good to sweat.
Felt like cursing out a few White women on separate occasions when they told me to move
They "need more space"
Never had that problem when dancing in my hometown
Where it's a quarter each of Asian Pacific American, Latinx, African American
And White people.
Got to class with my Warriors shirt on—my son said,
"Have to rep Oakland since it's the last year the team here."
We're in the middle of the NBA playoffs with 40 dancers and I'm the
Only one for Golden State—for real?
Are these folks from Oakland?
No need to translate the Latin Trap songs as I

Understand Spanish and learned how to
Cumbia in Texas where my husband is from.
Closer to my generation:
Sly Stone, ConFunkShun, E-40, Baby Bash,
Nef The Pharoah, S.O.B. x R.B.E., and H.E.R.
Closer to my son's generation all from
Vallejo now with population 122,000.
City good to grow up in but now
Police killing People of Color in record numbers.

Dancing once a week on Saturday morning used to be my therapy
Now my son Antonio says, "Mom, you should take class somewhere else."
Creature of habit in my middle age
Plus so convenient—too far to
Drive 50 miles roundtrip to
V-Town which taught me about
Resilience like how to stay on beat when
I can't remember the step.
How to give a eulogy at age 19 for my eldest brother
Who died of alcoholism at the age of 29.
How to make my way down a Soul Train line,
How to wear down a path in a
Shag carpet while Filipino friends taught me
How to Cha-Cha when I was
Fifteen years old like Antonio.
How to slow dance under a blue light basement party
Where we would dance off Earth Wind and Fire, Cameo, and
The Commodores—Remember "Brick House"?!?
No need to tell me between songs to
"Give someone a high five"
Save it for those women that need
Aerobic shoes
Choreographic directions
Air conditioning
More space
Just pump up the volume. . .
Like I said before—
I am from Vallejo.

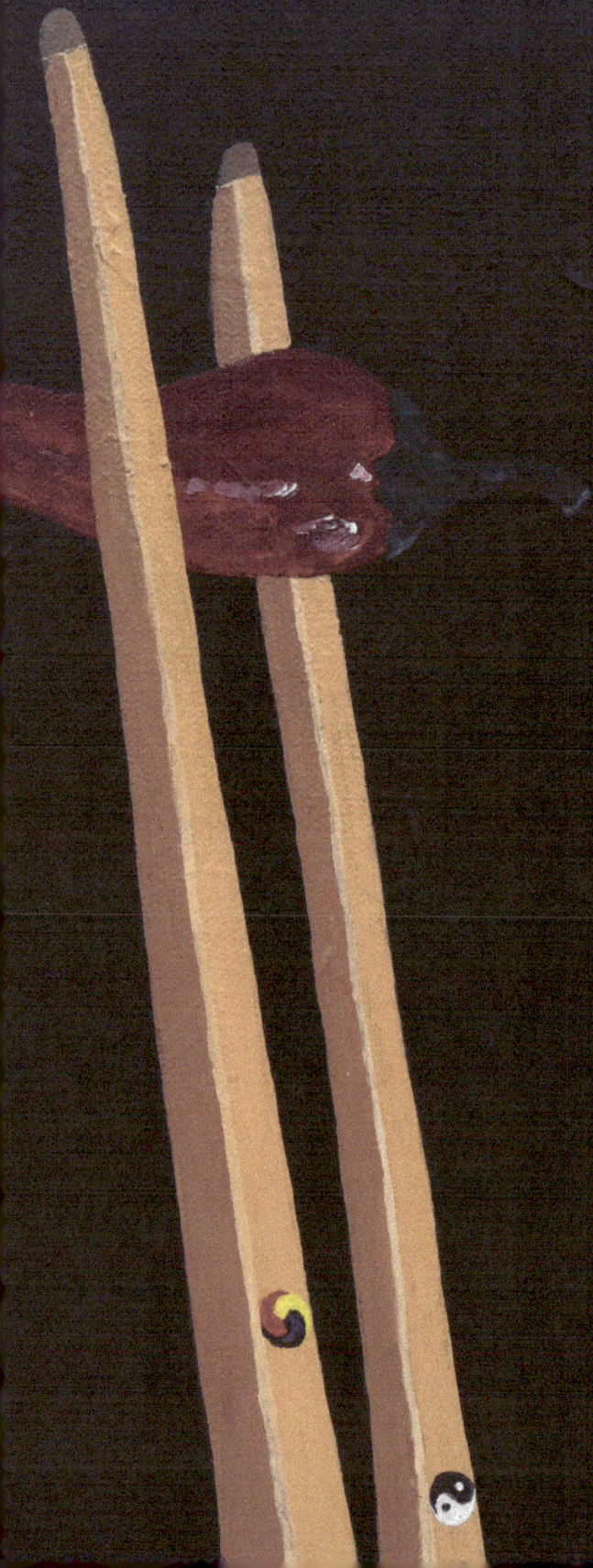

Exit 7 >>> Tennessee Street / Mare Island

This seventh exit introduces Tennessee Street, which had the only "walk-in" movie theater when I was growing up. It also leads into Mare Island, which was home of the Naval Shipyard; that industry propelled Vallejo until 1996 when it closed permanently. Vallejo is the surname of a Mexican general, so the legacy of Latinx people is in the name. This exit is devoted to Vallejoans with Latinx heritage.

One-Industry Town

Legend has it that General Vallejo lost one of his horses; it was found on Mare Island (Isla de la Yegua), the lifeblood of the City of Vallejo's economy for decades. Recently, I went to Mare Island and was amazed that I could drive directly onto the peninsula. When my father worked there for over 50 years, he had to drive over the causeway and civilians required clearance as it was a naval shipyard.

When my husband moved to Oakland with me from Texas in 1995, he said "Vallejo" with the Spanish pronunciation "Vy-aye-ho," not "Vuh-lay-oh," which is the way locals say it. We got into a humorous back-and-forth because I told him if he pronounced Northern California cities by the Spanish pronunciation, some people would not know which city he was talking about. Just like in Texas, locals tend to say "Am-uh-rilo" rather than "Ah-muh-ree-oh" for Amarillo, Texas. We chuckled about "Vacaville" (Cowtown) and "Manteca" (Lard), if one goes by the Spanish translation. Vallejo goes by "V-Town" and "Valley-Jo."

When I was growing up in the 1960s through 1980s, there was a sprinkling of Mexican families in the neighborhoods that fed into my elementary, junior, and high schools. When I go to Vallejo now, I am amazed by how much more of the population is Latinx. In fact, whenever we went on a day trip to Wine Country or Napa County, we always waited to drive back to Vallejo to stop for Mexican food. In junior high, our end-of-the-year field trip was to a Mexican restaurant called Mexico Lindo. When I think back, my teacher was Filipino and tri-lingual in English, Spanish, and Tagalog. Back then, there were two foreign language choices: French and Spanish. Thinking Spanish would be more useful, I continued with it in high school and college. I got a minor in Spanish while I was waiting for the impacted Occupational Therapy program at San Jose State University to accept me.

Working on "The Yard"

Working on Mare Island, or "The Yard" as my father would say, was sometimes generational. That is, government jobs in those times paid well and were very secure with a pension and other benefits for good work; this was not dependent on having a college degree. I had only gone to Mare Island once or twice when I was growing up, and I only remember passing the chapel there. When I went recently, I noted that there are some wineries, Touro University, and some film studios.

When I went to the Mare Island Museum, I felt like I was the only visitor at the time; it is run by volunteers and is small but mightily packed with information. On a wall, I was surprised to see a large wooden plaque noting "employees retired after 50 years of service to the fleet." "Herbert Ching" was listed as an "Electrical Mechanic" on May 3, 1993. His name was 19th on the list of 21. No wonder he looked bewildered when I left jobs after two or three years.

When I was growing up, the stereotype of Mexican people was the man with the sombrero sitting under a cactus with the implicit demeaning caption of "lazy." In truth, Mexican people work so hard and contribute much to our society. Mare Island was the source of the working-class nature of Vallejo, and the Mexican heritage of the city's namesake shows the history of Vallejo as part of "Alta California" in the 1800s. Vallejo has come full circle with the Latinx population continuing to grow. I never regret taking Spanish language courses as I can communicate with my family through marriage in a more meaningful way.

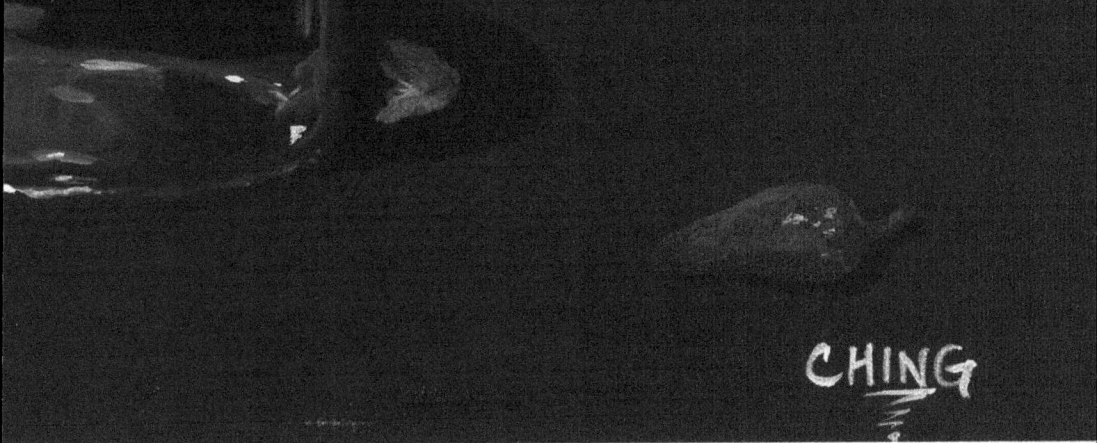

Still Life Chile

The chile pepper is indigenous to Mexico and because California used to be part of Mexico, I believe this acrylic painting I did several decades ago fits well with the vase of water. Being Korean, I used to enjoy spicy foods in my youth. However, as a middle-aged person I am "a lightweight" as I cannot handle too much heat in terms of taste, so do know that I am looking at my painting longingly now. I still like my food with a "little kick" to it occasionally—enjoy life!

Mixed Heritage (previous page)

Liking spicy food is part of being Korean and Mexican, for sure, and Chinese, especially food from the Hunan Province, which is depicted by the chopsticks and Yin Yang/balance symbols. "Yoon," "Ching," and "Diaz" are the surnames of my mother, father, and husband, respectively.

55

This poem speaks to my hope that I have earned every wrinkle, which reflects some wisdom along my life journey.

It is a cruel joke.
You get the senior discount only if you remember to go to the
Grocery Outlet on the second and fourth Tuesday mornings or Ross,
Tuesday evening.
I thought I would be taking Art classes when I was 12
Years away from getting full
Medicare and before
I started losing more of my eyesight—
I want to be able to see burnt sienna and
Lemon yellow.
Didn't know that I would
Get my doctorate otherwise I could
Not teach full-time at my job.
"Dr. Ching" my co-workers
call me before I can use the
"Dr" as a way
to encourage me
to finish the last lap
of my grueling
educational journey.
The only time anyone ever
Called me that
Was when I was eight years old and
My father would say,
"'Dr. Ching,' I need your good eyes to
take out my splinter."
Now my son is going to high
School and his middle-aged
Mom has a doctorate and
Has learned about confidence intervals,
Needs to publish in peer-reviewed journals
And knows she must wait a

Bit longer to dabble in
Umber and mauve.
Meanwhile, maybe my son will remind
Me when I can get the
Deep, deep
Discounts because
I surely do not remember
When to get carded to
Prove I am of age.

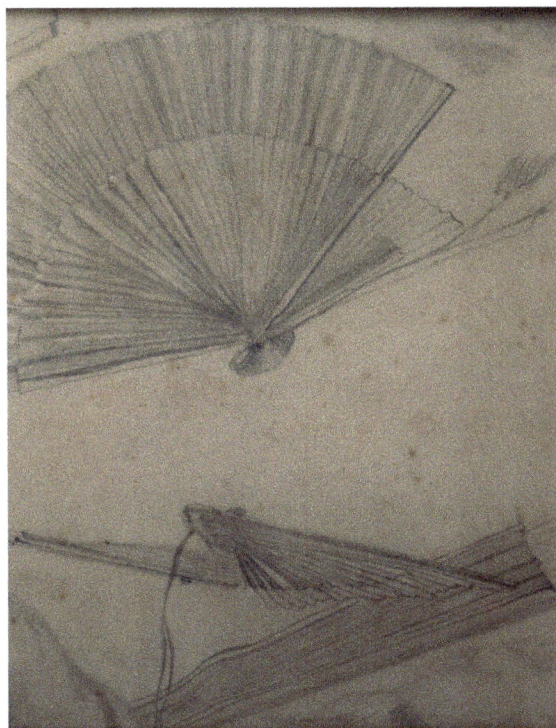

Fan of Fans

When I was in eleventh grade, I won a summer art scholarship at the Academy of Art in San Francisco. I stayed the summer in Oakland with my sister and brother-in-law and learned how to take the BART train and be in a "big city." This pencil drawing expresses the movement of the fan being made of fans, as the person holds the hypothetical fan with the backdrop of clouds.

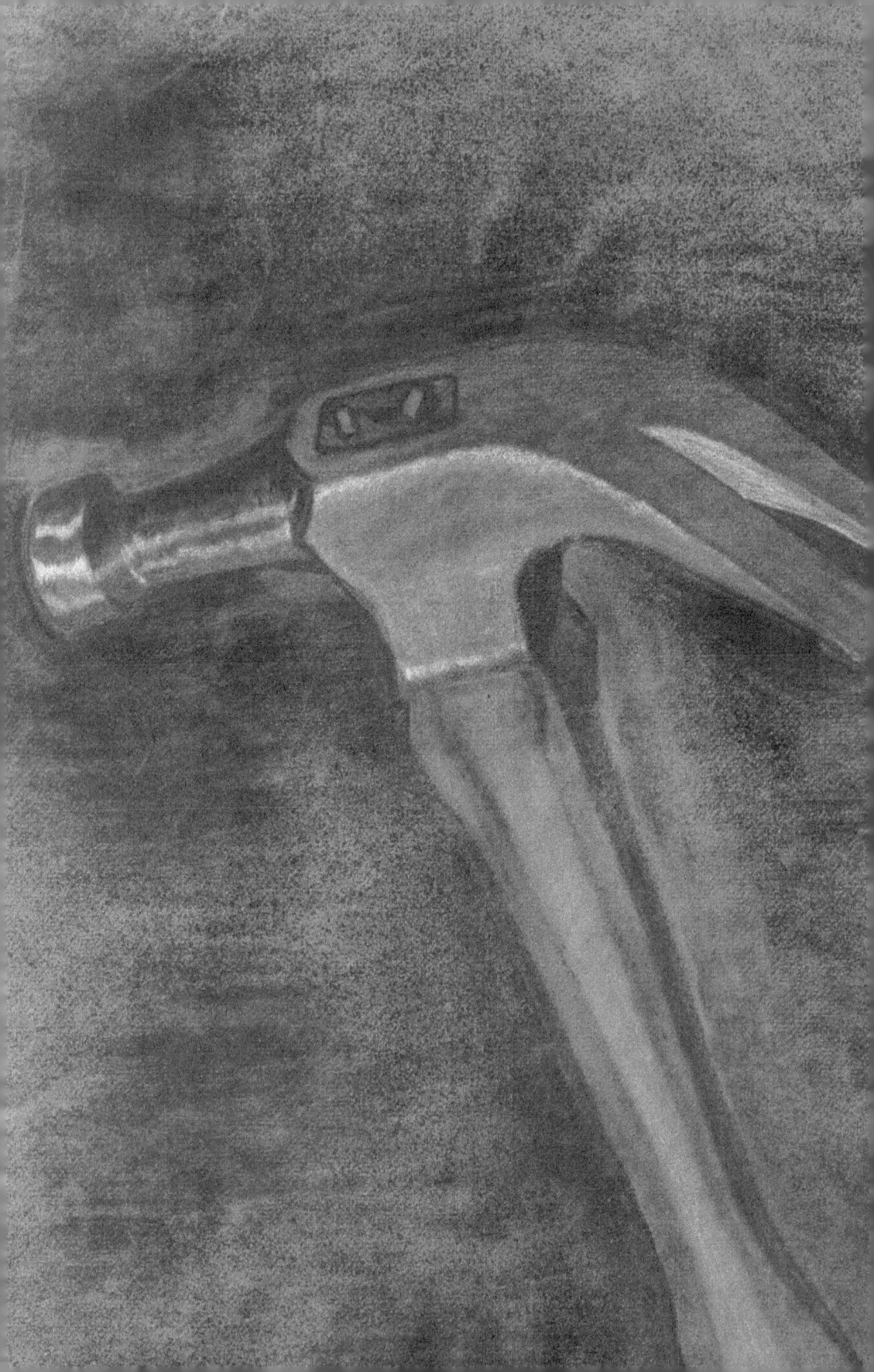

Exit 8 >>> Redwood Street

This eighth exit introduces Redwood Street, which is a thoroughfare to both Kaiser Hospital and Sutter Solano Hospital. This exit is devoted to Vallejoans with Filipinx heritage.

Kaiser Hospital and Trauma-Informed Care

For a small city, Vallejo, California has had three hospitals since the early 20th century: the Veteran's Administration (VA), Sutter Solano, and Kaiser Permanente. Because of the now-defunct Mare Island Naval Shipyard, two of the hospitals specifically served employees or military members and their families. Kaiser Hospital is off the Redwood Street exit located on Sereno Drive. Henry Kaiser was the Director of Kaiser Steel and headed up the early health maintenance organization (HMO) to provide cost-efficient care to injured steel workers and shipbuilders. When I was growing up, Vallejo General preceded the current Sutter Solano Hospital.

When I was a young college student, I had an appointment at Kaiser Vallejo and the nurse called my name off the appointment list. "Were you born in this hospital?" she asked quizzically. I responded affirmatively and asked her how she knew this fact. "Your chart is so thick," she replied with a knowing smile. On a recent trip to the Vallejo Historical and Maritime Museum, I found out that Kaiser Vallejo is still well-known for Proprioceptive Neuromuscular Facilitation (PNF), which is a treatment for those who have movement disorders. This treatment was developed by a physical therapist (PT) named Margaret Schott, who was based in the Kaiser Vallejo Rehabilitation Department. For those with muscular issues, the PNF technique is a set of movement-based patterns that assist the individual to gain more movement. Henry Kaiser's son had a disability and PNF benefitted him, so Kaiser opened the world-renown treatment for others, especially after World War II when veterans needed rehabilitation for war injuries.

Adverse Childhood Experiences (ACES) is well known in health care from an original study done in 1998 with Kaiser Permanente and the Centers for Disease Control and Prevention. The research revealed that early traumatic experiences affect health factors throughout the lifespan. The provision of trauma-informed care takes the ACEs into account. This is done by screening for early childhood trauma and factoring it into how care is provided. It is the alternative to treating each health issue in isolation from other issues that contribute to poor health outcomes.

Trauma-informed care has supplemented my thinking on how many health care professionals originate from Vallejo. I believe arts and sports can help those who suffer from various types of trauma. That is, after experiencing trauma, a healthy coping response is to create and mend the broken places in one's spirit. An unhealthy response is for the anger to erupt in destructive ways, inwardly as depression, or outwardly as expressing violence towards others. Resilience to trauma can take many creative forms, like fine art, writing, sports, theater arts, music, and so on. I would like to believe that is why I took up art, poetry, crafts, and writing—to heal some of the disjointed parts of my soul.

Courage in Nursing and Anti-Asian Racism

As everyone in health care knows, nurses are on the front lines of the COVID-19 pandemic. However, did you know that courage is one of the virtues in the profession of nursing? Filipinos have a long history in nursing. The Philippine Islands (P.I.) were colonized by the U.S., and the Philippines have provided nurses for the U.S. during shortages. Filipinos also have a long history with the Navy; at Subic Bay, Filipinos were cooks as they were not allowed to serve as sailors. Look at any Reserve Officers' Training Corps (ROTC) high school club on the West Coast and they are often filled with Filipino students.

As an occupational therapist, I know that my role on the health team does not require life or death decision making like nurses and physicians. In the profession of occupational therapy, Asian American Pacific Islander (AAPI) providers are often not considered underrepresented minorities (URM). However, Southeast Asians and Pacific Islanders definitely are underrepresented in our profession and in health care in general, because the AAPI tent is a large one, with a friend from Iran identifying herself as Asian. In occupational therapy, we use therapeutic activities to help patients or clients meet their goals. That is, occupational therapy is the art and science of healing the mind and body in a holistic manner. Fun fact: Little did I know that the high school teachers I write about in this book are coincidentally my art and biology teachers—the "Art and Science" of occupational therapy.

As an individual who identifies specifically as a Third Generation Korean Chinese American, the irony is not lost on me that every time the president consciously continues to say "Kung Flu" or "Chinese Virus" instead of Coronavirus or COVID-19, more anti-Asian racism will continue to take place in the U.S. For Asian American nurses, that may mean they are providing care for individuals who would have spit on them or denigrated them if they were on the streets, rather than in a health care setting.

If an Asian American nurse is in line at a grocery store wearing a coat, rather than personal protective equipment (PPE) like a mask in a hospital, they could be the target of a hate crime. Trust me—bigots do not take the time to differentiate between Asian nationalities. I have worked in health care and now health science academic settings since 1985. Well-intentioned personnel have mistaken me for other Asian American women on so many occasions, I have lost count. The pandemic has only exacerbated the ongoing disdain for Asian Americans in our society.

My understanding is that the letter "F" does not exist in Tagalog, which is the official language of the Philippines along with English, so "Filipino" is pronounced "Pilipino." Because of the many islands that compose P.I., numerous languages are spoken like Mindanao and Visayan, for example. The huge influence of Filipino culture cannot be underestimated in Vallejo. When I was growing up, the latest clothing, dance moves, and food were many times from Filipino students who went to P.I. or were well traveled and brought back the latest styles. Ask anyone of any race or ethnicity what "lumpia" is in Vallejo, and trust me—everyone knows and starts salivating.

Because the Philippines were also colonized by Spain, there are some common cultural components between Filipino and Mexican cultures. I swear that Tinikling, which is a Filipino dance that has dancers jump over bamboo sticks, and the Matachines Mexican dance, which has large wooden sticks dancers sidestep, look similar. Both share the beautiful rhythmic way folkloric dancers jump over the moving sticks that are tapped on the ground and used to give the beat.

One of the core values of Nursing is "Social Justice." There must be social justice for our nurses to be protected and equipped to do their essential work of fighting this pandemic war. Just as courage is a virtue in Nursing, let us have courage to support our nurses, nurse practitioners, physician assistants, physicians, and other frontline health care providers in whichever way we can.

Hard Work Hammer

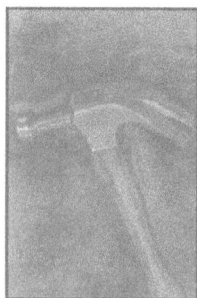

This charcoal drawing was sketched when I was in high school; it symbolizes the working-class City of Vallejo where I spent so many formative years. There is so much dignity and respect I feel for people who earn a living doing blue-collar work. "Essential Workers" are often people like my family, through genetics and also marriage, who are denied their worth as human beings because they do not have a privileged status in our society. Collectively, through their hard work and determination, our ancestors built this country, be it the bridges, railroads, buildings, highways—you name it. They deserve better in life and in the history books.

Table Tiger Lilies

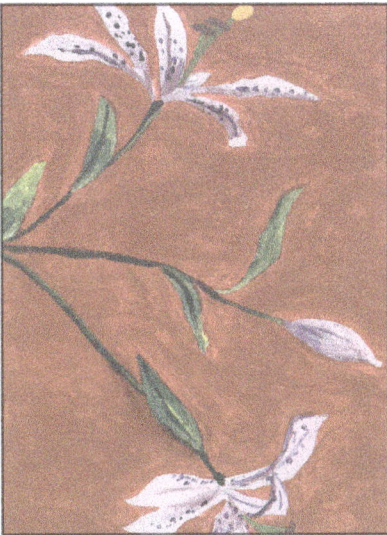

I lived near a historically Black university (HBU) named Huston-Tillotson when I resided in Austin, Texas. It was located in East Austin, which was also the home of a large Mexican American community, as Black and Brown people lived east of Interstate Highway 35 or IH 35. Due to gentrification, my understanding now is that East Austin has more coffee shops than Black bookstores or taquerias like it had when we lived there from the late 1980s to the mid 1990s.

I took an acrylic painting class with a Chicano artist who had his art studio in East Austin, and this is the still life I painted in his class. Whether it is a tiger or a tiger lily, I am always drawn to tigers, which symbolize beauty, wisdom, and strength in my view.

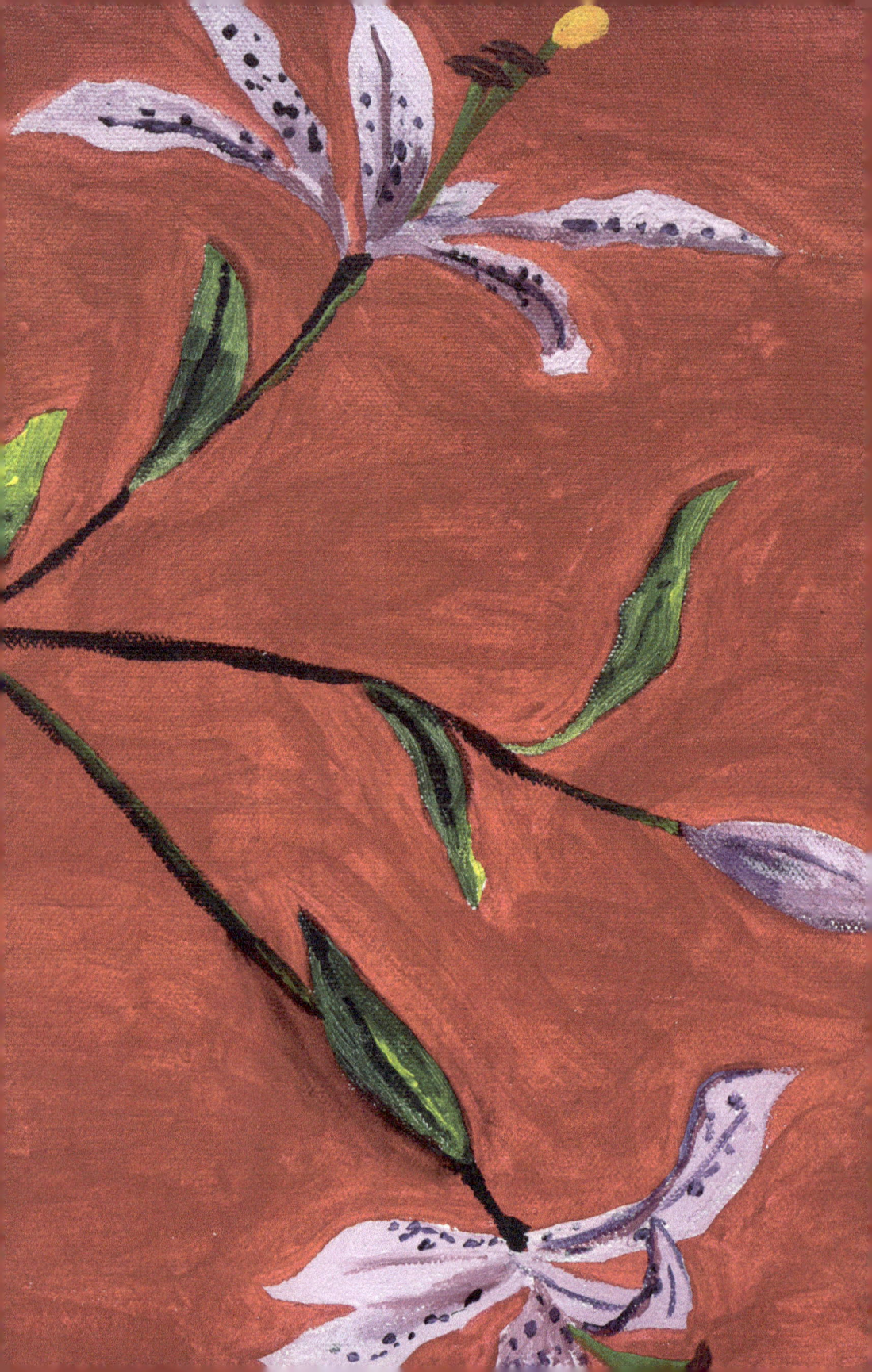

No Lipstick

I quit wearing lipstick—
It colors the inside of my mask burgundy.
Feels like Halloween as I see
Fellow Oakland dwellers
With masks on
During the Covid-19 pandemic
"Trick or Treat" I feel like saying. . .
"Trick" is long lines
"Treat" is toilet paper
"Trick" is not being able to visit
My brother at the VA
"Treat" is that he has
Given his lungs a rest as he cannot smoke now
"Trick" is we had to cancel our Spring Break
Trip to Texas
"Treat" is my
"Love Letter to Laredo"
Was published in the *Laredo Morning Times*
Perhaps by the end of this
Mask-wearing shelter-in-place period
I will smile widely wearing
Revlon's Superlustrous
#640 Blackberry
Glistening
On my bare face.

Exit 9 >>> Redwood Parkway West

This ninth exit introduces Redwood Parkway, which has Latinx day laborers on the side of the road looking for work. This exit is devoted to Vallejoans with Mexican heritage.

When I was growing up, the Redwood Parkway exit did not exist. Redwood Street was the exit for the Fairgrounds and Lake Chabot, which was developed and turned into Marine World and later Six Flags Discovery Kingdom. Six Flags is an amusement park that originated in Texas and is so named because the state was under the six flags of Spain, France, Mexico, Republic of Texas, the Confederate States, and finally the United States of America.

Love Letter to Laredo

The following was published in a slightly different form on April 16, 2020 in the Laredo Morning Times.

People will be fined $1,000 if they are in public without a mask or face covering. Say what? The City Council of Laredo, Texas decided to enact stringent measures to discourage the spread of COVID-19. I am worried about how low-income individuals can afford to pay the hefty fine or have access to a face mask, but I understand the intent of the measure. I am a health professional and professor and have been traveling to Laredo since 1989 as my husband is a native Laredoan.

According to the 2010 Census, Laredo has the most "homogeneous" zip codes in the U.S., with 95.2% of the population being Hispanic or Latino and the majority of Laredoans identifying as Mexican American or Mexican. Stopping the spread of Coronavirus in Laredo is vitally important so as not to overwhelm the two major hospitals. In contrast to my husband, I was born in Vallejo, California, which has the most "heterogeneous" zip codes in the U.S., which reflects the racial and ethnic diversity there. I am a proud Third Generation Korean Chinese American from a working-class neighborhood. I lived on Magazine

Street, which means something to you if you are a musical fan of West Coast hip hop—it is the street where E-40 grew up.

When I shop at small mom and pop stores in downtown Laredo, customers say, "Dónde está ésa cosa?" or "Where is that thing?" Many times the owners of these stores are Korean. The customers think I own the shop since I am Asian. I reply, "No trabajo aquí" or "I don't work here." When I return, I good-naturedly tell my husband that I have been racially profiled. Instead of saying, "Asiático" or "Asian," Spanish-speakers often say "Chinos," which literally means "Chinese people." Korea and China are countries with their own distinct languages, histories, and cultures. Mexico and Brazil are also countries with their own distinct languages, histories, and cultures, and no one would ever dream of calling all Latinos "Brazilian," for example. Instead of getting offended, I just smile as technically I am half Chinese and half Korean. I cannot ever get too mad at Laredoans. When we go to Laredo we stay with my mother-in-law, who sometimes affectionately calls me "m'ija" or "daughter," and who is 89 years old but still remembers my birthday, Mother's Day, and even our wedding anniversary.

Laredoans sometimes call tacos "mariachis" and when you order "wines," it may not be alcoholic beverages but rather "wieners" or hot dogs. This South Texas city is rich in culture, but it may be one of the cities hardest hit economically by the COVID-19 shuttering of businesses. I sent hand-sewn masks to our family in Laredo to stay safe and meet the city directive to wear masks in public places. Laredo is our second home and is our family. We hope we will be able to visit by the holiday season. Viva Laredo, Tejas!

Hinge Joint

In this poem I use a metaphor to anchor the tragedy of the murder of George Floyd.

Ask any athlete, worker, person—the
Importance of the
Knee
Who knew that the
Same hinge joint
Which with Kap
Could protest
Would be the very
Same hinge joint
Which would
Drain the life
From George
And spark a
Movement
The definition of "Hinge"
Is "a moveable joint or mechanism on which
A door, gate, or lid swings as it opens and closes or
Which connects linked objects."
I pray that this
Hinge opens the
Door to structural change in the U.S.
And closes the Door
On the legacy of
Racism

June 2, 2020

Exit 10 >>> Columbus Parkway / Napa / Novato

This tenth exit introduces Columbus Parkway, which connects with freeways to Napa (Napa County) and Novato (Marin County). This exit is devoted to Vallejoans with African American heritage.

Country Club Crest

George Floyd was buried on June 9, 2020 in Houston, Texas. I observed his passing as the legacy of structural racism, where African Americans were segregated to the Country Club Crest, or "The Crest," which continues to be home to many African Americans in Vallejo today. There is a large retaining wall on the right-hand side of the freeway that blocks the Crest neighborhood from view. Because of the Great Migration of African Americans from 1915 to 1970 from the South, many of my friends who identified as Black had family in Georgia, Louisiana, Texas, and so on. I would not see my teenage peers because they would be sent "Down South" for the summer; their families wanted them to be with relatives there to absorb some of the culture at least for two or three months.

African American culture is so integral to the essence of Vallejo. The Black Panthers had a Chapter in Vallejo, and The Black Muslim Bakery came from Oakland to sell fresh-baked bread to us in the 1970s. Sly Stone is from Vallejo, and Sly and the Family Stone was a racially diverse musical band that was groundbreaking at the time. The irony of the Columbus Parkway exit is that the Crest is the last Vallejo neighborhood on the way to Napa where "White Flight" occurred; White people moved to Napa, Novato, Santa Rosa, and beyond to get away from the People of Color in Vallejo.

My high school badminton team was very racially diverse and we had to play Vintage High (get it—Napa is known for its wine growing). Even at that young high school age, we sort of bristled and became more guarded because of the way we were treated in Napa. In my experience, People of Color, especially African Americans, have required antennae for racism or discriminatory acts. Those antennae helped everyone on the team stay safe. We were made up of Latinas, Asians, Whites, and

African Americans and were on high alert when we walked into their gymnasium.

The Wine Train and Pet Therapy

I was hoping the discrimination from White people in Napa was ancient history, but the Wine Train discriminatory incident happened in 2015. African American passengers, on a train where one can sample Napa Valley wines, were kicked off for being "too loud," even though other passengers were louder but were not Black. This incident is not unusual and I was not surprised when I read about it, even though Napa Valley is the second highest tourist attraction in California after Disneyland.

As a professor at a health science university, I forget that the majority of my colleagues at work are White and female; often, they do not know the historical context of People of Color and health systems. For example, part of my work is supervising graduate students working on their capstone project, which is our version of a practical and much shorter dissertation. A well-meaning White student asked my approval to bring her dog to a site where I supervised students working with older adults, primarily African American and from the Southern part of the U.S. Pet therapy is the practice of bringing a pet to a site for the patients or clients to interact with to build rapport with the pet and generate positive emotions. Ultimately, I had to tell my colleagues that I did not believe bringing a pet would generate positive emotions with the population at the site for the majority of the clients there.

"Why not?" my colleagues asked. I told them that I would be making some generalizations and each individual might respond differently; however, growing up in a predominantly Black neighborhood, I observed many things. First, for many People of Color, dogs served a dual purpose. Dogs were pets but mainly served as watchdogs—protectors of property by being menacing through bark or with bite. Moreover, people in low-income neighborhoods do not have disposable income for the dog's immunizations, flea care, food, and so on. Therefore, the dog has to "earn its keep," so to speak. One White male colleague said, "Some Black people are afraid of dogs." No lie. Plus, during the Civil Rights

Movement, police released dogs on peaceful protesters, so there is more history of dogs being threatening. Finally, I told my colleagues privately and with goodwill, "If the student has a rabbit or hamster, she can complete her pet therapy capstone at the site." Unfortunately, she did not and had a large German Shepard. I often wish I could offer a health science course on the historical context of People of Color and health care in the U.S.

Serving Students During the COVID-19 Pandemic

The following is an article I sent to an occupational therapy newsletter regarding serving our most vulnerable students during the COVID-19 Pandemic.

Let's face it—students of color in our profession have been a vulnerable population even prior to the COVID-19 global pandemic. To be clear, our classes are generally held in-person; however, because of the need to physically distance ourselves, we have been given temporary status of offering courses online. I identify as a faculty of color and strive for inclusive online strategies to decrease stress and engage all Occupational Therapy (OT) students, knowing that these strategies are particularly salient for students of color.

1. **Keep course communications to a minimum.** I make a weekly announcement in Canvas, which is our learning platform at my university. Early Sunday evening I generally make the announcement in order to have the students' full attention.

2. **Try and project positivity while imparting information.** Rather than stating a "To-Do" list of requirements, I write "Friendly Reminders" instead.

3. **Use praise freely.** Recently I wrote in my announcement that "I was pleased with your literature reviews." This does not mean you cannot give constructive feedback, but it just sets a pleasant tone for the online conversation.

4. **State alternatives for meeting the technological demands of the online class.** Before students gave their online group presentations, I noted that if anyone had technical problems, like audio or screen-sharing issues, I would simply grade their written papers they already posted and not penalize their group grade. They remarked in the chat feature, "Thank you so much, Dr. Ching!"

5. **Infuse appropriate therapeutic-use-of-self bits of humor.** Because my practice area is mental health since 1985, I teach courses similarly to how I facilitate groups. That is, each class is like an essay with a beginning, middle, and end. As a colleague remarked, "Beth, you are so into icebreakers and closures!" Recently at the conclusion of a course, I summarized and told the students that I was grateful for their participation, flexibility, and resilience during these difficult days. At the very end of the class, this middle-aged professor pretended to drop the imaginary microphone and said loudly, "Peace Out!"

During this COVID-19 "Shelter-in-place" Period (as it is called in California), we are all under so much stress. In my phone conversations with students of color, I have noted that many of them have to return home to live with multi-generational family members, so they are especially concerned about keeping older adults in the household free from the virus. Because African American and Latinx people affected by COVID-19 are disproportionately unable to "socially distance" due to being essential workers, students return home and may need to "fill in" for a parent to help homeschool younger siblings, help with the family income or business, or take another familial role, leaving less time for their student role.

Because of the Digital Divide, having adequate broadband capability is not an option. Moreover, even doing a PowerPoint presentation is challenging given that Microsoft charges an annual licensing fee for that feature. I have observed students using Google Docs and downloading free graphics for slides to compensate for not having access to PowerPoint. When a textbook is required for class, I list the most recent edition in the course syllabus; however, in reality, I know that many students of color reference the topic and have to use an outdated edition because they cannot afford the newest edition, even to lease, which is a cheaper option than buying the textbook outright.

Given our current COVID-19 situation, perhaps Telehealth has become a reality for occupational therapy practitioners. I sincerely hope these online learning strategies will be helpful not just in academia but also in practice settings. These are strategies with the aim to eliminate health disparities to achieve health equity for all. In summary, "Peace Out, Esteemed Colleagues!" Stay safe and well.

On Solidarity & "Strength in Numbers"

You Don't Know Me

It finally happened—last week, a man hurled Anti-Asian profanities at me when I was walking home. Honestly, it's not that important what he shouted, but more importantly the fact that he was a young brother of color, specifically African American. Honestly, I was not surprised by the "All you Asians can suck my d–!" since I was born in 1962 and have heard so many racial epithets and have been racially bullied before I even had language to explain what happened to me. Anti-Asian sentiments hurt the most coming from People of Color.

Being an Asian American woman is being in a no-win situation. Here is how I had to respond to the racially-charged incident. I was walking past the man on the sidewalk where he was on his bicycle, and I walked about 50 feet before he started shouting. Right then I knew he was a coward, otherwise he would of said something to my face and not let me walk a ways out. When I heard him screaming, I just kept walking with my back to him, but I gave him the finger with both my raised hands. He must have seen my gestures because he started screaming with more voracity. I did not look back but replied with a profanity in return which was basically, "Get your hating a– out of my neighborhood!" If I were not a middle-aged Asian woman, I could have been more therapeutic by saying, "I know you were raised better than that." However, because of stereotypes of older Asian women being quiet and not fighting back, I felt compelled to dispel that myth by shouting a profanity as loudly as I could in case he tried to run up on me.

You see, he did not know me. As an Asian American growing up in a Black neighborhood, I learned how to observe people. In my view, African Americans often have to develop an authenticity antennae for survival, and I did too as a Korean Chinese American where the only other people of my ethnicities were my siblings. If I said some fighting words to someone, then I had better get ready to defend myself as I would not be able to hide in a crowd of my peers because there were no others to defend us.

No one is trying to kill me or cause me harm because of the color of my skin, so I strongly believe, "Black Lives Matter." Colorism is real. Let me tell you that almond-shaped eyes being a target is a result of White Supremacy also. Wearing a mask while Black is a thing. Wearing a mask while Asian is also a thing. I cannot disguise the shape of my eyes, nor would I want to. By the way, I did report the Anti-Asian incident on the STOP AAPI HATE reporting form. This information needs to be tracked in order for there to be data as evidence to get funding to combat Anti-Asian racism. I am part of the statistics now. As a proud Native Vallejoan and now Oaklander, I follow the NBA Warriors Team. Their motto is "Strength in Numbers." Now is the time for all people to fight systemic racism and for People of Color to be in solidarity with one another so that our solidarity is our strength in numbers as well.

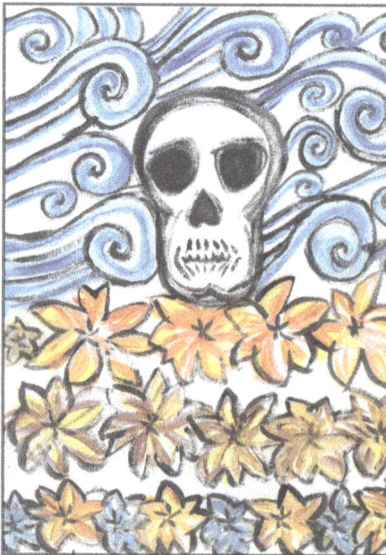

Calavera Plumeria

Latinx Legacy is the Latinx Affinity Group that sponsored a Mexican Día de Muertos paint night at my work, and I meant to paint the traditional marigolds associated with the honoring of ancestors, which the instructor painted as an example. All my flowers ended up looking like plumeria more associated with Hawaii, so I let them be.

Thoughts on Cultural Appropriation

"Don't wear that, Mom," my son told me after I sewed a cotton beige and blue patterned jacket. "Why not?" I replied as I was just about to try it on and was so pleased with how it turned out. I looked at the pattern again, and I said, "It looks like an African print, right?" He gave me a knowing head nod, and I said, "No worries." I gifted the jacket to my niece who is biracial African American / Asian American and smart, talented, and beautiful. I had bought the fabric at Payless Drug Store on 51st Street in Oakland in the 1990s when they had a fabric section. I get it and I understand how the dominant culture often appropriates and profits from non-dominant culture or from People of Color.

That said, the current strict codes of who gets to write, speak, or wear "culture" is puzzling to me perhaps because I do come from Vallejo. For example, I wrote a piece about Thanksgiving, and I realized that my mother used to say she was "fixin'" to do something—spelled out, it would be "fixing to," which meant she was planning to do an activity. In Black English, I suspect that would be what my elementary school classmates would shorten to say "I fin' to go to the store and get some candy." I neglected to mention that my mother moved to many places in the U.S. so I do not know exactly the origins of how she came by "fixin'."

When I was a teenager, good-looking boys were "Foin" instead of "Fine"—with the "Foin..." stretched out as long as an exhaled breath. "He was 'foin' and didn't know it which is the best kind" my neighbor said, which meant that the young man was handsome but did not act pretentious. I realize that I have had to codeswitch for as long as I can remember. You see how confusing it is to interpret ways of speaking for this middle-aged, Third Generation, Asian American who grew up in a predominantly Black neighborhood? I do what we all have to do for my work as I have to speak Standard English. When I am with people who really know me and who identify as African American, I feel freer to speak what is on my mind, which does not always come out in Standard English. In my experience, most African Americans have an authenticity antennae as a survival skill. I have known that for a long time; however, if I were with friends who identify as African American, we could just do shorthand by saying, "I bin' knew that."

In the 1980s, I remember the Ben Davis pants, Pendleton wool shirts buttoned all the way up the neck, white tank tops, and black "Winos" shoes being the style popularized from "Cholos" or Mexican Americans especially associated with Lowrider car culture. The women's version of the Winos were "Mary Jane" shoes—sometimes the black canvas shoes were machine embroidered with colorful flowers. The Winos and Mary Jane shoes were made in China as they were originally inexpensive, martial arts-type shoes. I never had a problem when seeing people who were not Chinese wearing shoes made in China back then or now. Especially now, since so many athletic and basketball shoes in particular are made in China. Not long ago, I went to a workshop on how to embroider taught by a member of the organization where my husband works. The teacher was Yucatecan from Mexico, and she brought each sewer a Mexican wedding-style blouse to embroider around the neckline and hem. I embroidered the standard flowers and I added a yin-yang symbol of my Chinese heritage. Unfortunately, by the current set of appropriation standards, I must leave my embroidered blouse packed away since I could be accused of cultural appropriation if I wear it. This just makes me feel downtrodden when I had felt so exhilarated when I was learning to embroider the stitches.

I have always loved Chinese brocade material, especially in red. The color red has deep meaning for Chinese people as it signifies luck, and the deep crimson shade accentuates my skin tone. When I was growing up, if I wore a Mandarin collar red Chinese brocade blouse or top, one of three things would happen to me: 1) I would be called "Chink" or "Chinamen"; 2) People would assume I worked at a Chinese restaurant; or 3) Someone would shout, "Go back to where you come from!" I must tell you that this disdain would not only come from Whites but other People of Color (POC), which hurt the most because I had expected more from my POC brothers and sisters. In my view, this is how Anti-Asian behavior shows up. I would have been proud to wear Asian clothing, but I was always made to feel shame around being singled out for wearing traditional clothing from my culture. Therefore, I am puzzled when my brothers and sisters who are People of Color and not Asian American or Pacific Islanders are quick to point out cultural appropriation when they themselves have tattoos of Chinese characters or have large jade necklaces of Buddha. I honestly do not have an issue with it other than the obvious one of hypocrisy.

When I moved back to California from Texas in 1995, I had picked up saying "Y'all" from being in Texas. I hadn't planned on it—it just stuck as I had lived in Austin from 1989 to 1995. It made sense just like in Spanish with its plural form of "You" being "Usted" (Ud.), which translates to "Ustededs" (Uds.) or "You all" or "Y'all." Being an occupational therapist leading groups, I would have many occasions to say "Y'all" when giving directions. At one of my places of work, I said, "Y'all" and I was ridiculed by my co-workers in front of all the clients I was teaching. The people who shamed me were from a diversity of ethnic backgrounds. I guess as an Asian American, it was taboo for me to say "Y'all." I had to start saying "You guys," which I loathe, so I settled on "Folks." Being Asian American is being in a no-win situation in the U.S. I feel damned if I do and damned if I don't. As I get older, I feel even more invisible, which I didn't think was actually possible.

I teach a course entitled, "Health Promotion and Wellness." I was so honored reading an anonymous comment on my course evaluation from a student which read, "Dr. Ching is a wonderful teacher. In less capable hands, this course could be considered cultural appropriation." That is, some of the topics include Mindfulness-based Stress Reduction (MBSR), Chinese Medicine, Yoga, etc. Being present in the moment or "mindfulness" has its origins in Buddhism, acupuncture and acupressure comes from China, yoga which is a spiritual practice is from India, and I cannot imagine how much South Asian people might be horrified of White people doing "Goat Yoga." I believe our ancestors from all our cultures were wise, and the topics we cover in the course come from ancient wisdom based on research which was available to our peoples at the time, i.e. writing down observations over thousands of years in the case of Chinese Medicine.

Western society has re-packaged and re-framed our peoples' ancient wisdom and ancestral knowledge and profited from "anecdotal Folk remedies" and re-purposed these to "evidence-based practice," which is how the ancestral knowledge is transcribed into peer-reviewed journal research and transfers hands. If we know the context and are respectful of a peoples' history and do not use it for personal monetary gain, I do not take issue with an exchange between cultures. Culture is not static, and we have benefited from the intermingling. I like spaghetti, which is Italian, but Marco Polo got the idea of pasta from going to China, which is the Country of Origin of hand-cut noodles.

Can you picture how common it is for people to put their hands over their temples by the corner of their eyes and pull their eyelids back as the universal derogatory sign language for demeaning "slant eyes" or Asians as a People? It always amazes me that when people are called out for doing this, their defense is that they did not think it was offensive. I have heard someone close (not Chinese) say that her mother made her pony-tail so tight that it gave her "Chinese eyes." People know about colorism where fairer or whiter skin is more valued due to White Supremacy; however, people do not give credence to the fact that East Asian people have been brainwashed to believe that "round eyes" are more beautiful also due to White Supremacy. In parts of Asia, people get "the eye surgery." I suspect some K-Pop singers get both the whitening cream and the round-eye treatment.

When I was taunted and bullied as a child and young woman with "How can you see anything out of those beady, slant eyes?" I had no comeback. Now that you know a bit of my history, believe me when I say, "I can see more out of these almond-shaped eyes than you ever will" to those Bigots who hurled taunts and who were emboldened by being in a group, acting like they were all bad—how much courage are you showing when you have a herd mentality against a lone child? Not being on the dichotomy of Black or White allows me to see the beauty of all our cultures—one just needs to be mindful. Remember that Mexican blouse I embroidered? I expressed my sadness of not being able to wear the blouse I embroidered to my Latinx friend. Do you know what she said? She looked at me dead in the eye and said, "Beth, just wear it—you're not Mexican but you are a great ally. White women wear whatever the hell they want and they don't give a shit!" If I get the blouse out of the box and get the courage to wear it, I guess if I get called out, I will just say, "It was given to me by a friend." Technically that is true as my embroidery teacher is a friend.

I am grateful to Vallejo because I am proud of where I come from and I wanted to give homage to how we were able to get along with one another in my hometown. I write this as police are still killing our youth of color in record numbers. If Vallejo in its racial diversity is a microcosm of the U.S., is there hope to abolish structural racism in our Country? Truly that is my desire. When I was in my 30s in the Honolulu airport returning to the Continental U.S., the airline ticket staff asked me, "Sure you're going to the Mainland?" That is, he looked at me as an Asian American with my Latinx husband and thought we were mistakenly headed in the wrong line. This is the first time I had ever felt like the assumption was that I belonged where I was; I fit in somewhere. As soon as I responded, I am sure the staff person could tell I had a Mainland accent, but for a split second, I belonged. With my story coming from Vallejo as an Korean Chinese American from a predominantly Black neighborhood married to a Latino with our son being Asian Latinx, I do not fit anywhere, but I fit everywhere.

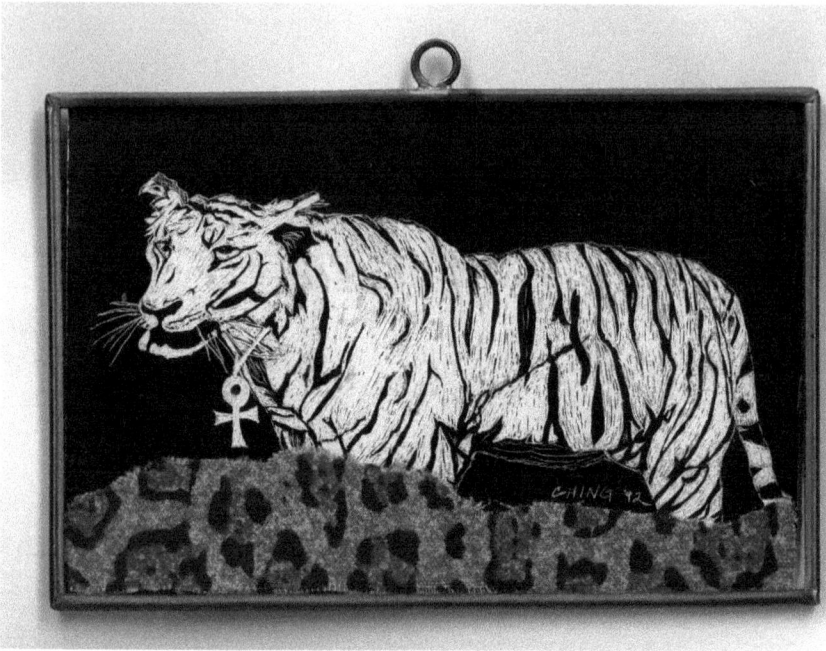

Year of the Woman Tiger

The tiger wears an ankh, which is an Egyptian symbol of life; it also represents the female gender. I "burned out" working in acute psychiatric facilities when I lived in Austin, Texas; at the time, I worked at an ethnic arts store and also for a Latinx arts organization. A Latina artist from that organization showed me how to use linocut, which is what this is, plus leopard flannel fabric.

My sister Miriam and I are twelve years apart and are both tigers on the Chinese astrological calendar. She has lived in Korea and told me that traditionally, women born under a more passive animal sign like "rabbit," for example, are more valued. I did this piece to reflect how strong we are as women of color and to symbolize rejecting patriarchy by being proud women tigers.

Past-Future: Aara Amidi-Nouri–PRESENTE!

My dear friend, colleague, and mentor Aara Amidi-Nouri passed away too soon in April 2020. She was a true co-conspirator and a proud nurse, educator, and organizer. We always spoke about the need for People of Color to show up for one another in our different struggles. I cannot think of a better moment than now to say, "Tu lucha es mi lucha" or "Your fight is my fight."

Girlfriend, I am taking your passing away real hard
I have too many tears and stories to bear
Angel Warrior
Your friendship enveloped me in a cozy blanket
Let me just tell about the time
When we had to take the MindTime
Thinking Assessment at work
Remember, where it was like a horoscope for
What kind of thinker you are?
That is, what guides your decisions?
Lenses of the Past, Present, or Future
Like Dicken's "A Christmas Carol" but instead of ghosts
There were color-coded stickers
For me, I scored Past and Present
I think of the context of an issue and then the current reality.
For you, you scored Past and Future
You think of the history of an issue just like me but then you envision the future.
Aara, you said that was probably why
You got into so much trouble
Since you contextualized the situation at hand,
But were driven to see the outcomes and possibilities
Being impatient with the present with its
Challenges, barriers, bureaucracy
No wonder you got frustrated with the current state of the
Social Determinants of Health and Health Disparities
Poor Health Outcomes for People of Color
Laughingly, you remarked, "I understand the Past—
Can't we just skip the Present and
Get to a better Future?"

You envisioned high school youth of color
Using their junior and senior years in dual enrollment for college
Credits so that they could have a
BSN degree after 2 years at
Community College to be a Nurse
They could graduate earlier and start helping
Their families financially right away.
The Thinking Assessment was wrong—
You have given us a Present
By Gifting us with your Vision for a Just Future.
Aara Amidi-Nouri—PRESENTE!

April 4, 2020

References

About Kaiser Permanente. (2015, March 5). "Margaret 'Maggie' Knott, pioneer physical therapist." https://about.kaiserpermanente.org/our-story/our-history/margaret-maggie-knott-pioneer-physical therapist

Burke Harris, N. (2018). *The deepest well: Healing the long-term effects of childhood adversity.* Houghton Mifflin Harcourt.

Ceniza Choy, C. (2003). *Empire of care: Nursing and migration in Filipino American history.* Duke University Press.

Ching, E., & Ammon, A. (2020). "Navigating the tide: Health science student and faculty of color academic experiences." *Diversity & Equality in Health and Care,* 16(4), 101-106. Doi: 10.36648/2049-5471.17.1.199

Eligon, J. (2017). "Does race matter in America's most diverse ZIP codes?" *The New York Times.*

McGriff-Payne, S. (2012). *African Americans in Vallejo.* Arcadia Publishing.

Orpilla, M. (2005). *Filipinos in Vallejo.* Arcadia Publishing.

Poblete, P.N. (2018). *A better place: A memoir of peace in the face of tragedy.* Nothing But The Truth Publishing, L.L.C.

Riley, B. (2017). *Lower Georgia Street: California's forgotten Barbary Coast.* Arcadia Publishing.

Vallejo Naval and Historical Museum. https://www.vallejomuseum.org

Veronica, N.A. (2007). *World War II shipyards by the bay.* Arcadia Publishing.

Vickers, M. (2017). *You can't return home except through photographs & memory.* Marquis Publishing.

Wikipedia: The free encyclopedia. https://www.wikipedia.org

Wilkerson, I. (2010). *The warmth of other suns: The epic story of America's great migration.* Random House, Inc.

Acknowledgments

To both my husband and son Antonio who have sustained me—I say, "Te quiero mucho!" To Miriam, Matthew, Ernest, and Belvin, I am indebted to you as my sister, brothers, and brother-in-law who have raised and supported me. To my editor Valerie Haynes-Perry, I thank you for the Writing Circle Sisters and profound encouragement to "Write the book I want to read." To Nguyen and Rabbit Roar, I could not have done this without you. To Jai Arun Ravine, thank you for making this book beautiful. To my departed compañera Aara Amidi-Nouri, I rededicate myself to this work for health equity for all. To the families of those murdered by the police in Vallejo, I wish you justice. Finally, to all the Vallejoans, I see you in the 707!

About the Author

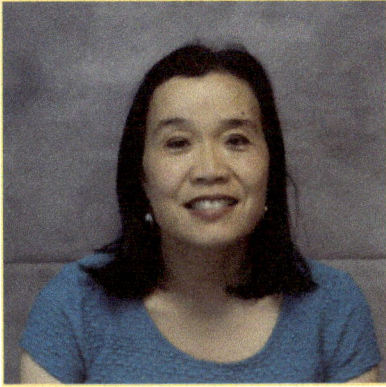

Elizabeth "Beth" Ching, OTD, M.Ed., BSOT, OTR/L, Associate Professor, Samuel Merritt University (SMU), is a Third Generation Korean Chinese American born in Vallejo, California and has been an occupational therapist since 1985. Beth has been committed to working with underserved populations throughout her career. She has presented at the National Conference on Race and Ethnicity in Higher Education (NCORE) about reducing health disparities and mentoring Black, Indigenous, People of Color (BIPOC) youth to enter the health professions. She also held the SMU Faculty Diversity Coordinator position in the Office of Diversity and Inclusion. Dr. Ching has published in the *Journal of Cultural Diversity, Journal of Occupational Therapy Education, Journal of Diversity and Equality in Health and Care*; she has co-authored "Psychosocial and Cognitive Issues Affecting Therapy" in *Neurorehabilitation for the Physical Therapist Assistant* (2021). Dr. Ching was honored to receive the 2021 Faculty of the Year Award at SMU.

www.ingramcontent.com/pod-product-compliance
Lightning Source LLC
Chambersburg PA
CBHW052120030426
42335CB00025B/3075